THE ANAESTHESIA VIVA

VOLUME 2

Physics, Measurement, Clinical Anaesthesia, Anatomy & Safety

Mark Blunt
John Urquhart

With contributions from Ian Driver

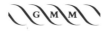

© 1997
Greenwich Medical Media
137 Euston Road
London
NW1 2AA

ISBN 1 900151 405

First Published 1997
Reprinted 2000

Printed in Great Britain by
Ashford Colour Press

PREFACE

1996 has seen a fundamental change in postgraduate training of anaesthetists. In place of the traditional 'apprentice system' without a clear start and finish there is now a structured course of training, under the auspices of the Royal College of Anaesthetists, consisting of two years at Senior House Officer (SHO) level and four years as a specialist registrar (SpR) with a new two part examination (Primary and Final) for the Diploma of Fellowship of the Royal College of Anaesthetists (FRCA). The new Primary examination consists of three elements, multiple choice questions (MCQs), a set of sixteen objectively structured clinical examinations (OSCEs) and two Vivas. Viva One covers physiology, pharmacology and statistics and Viva Two covers physics, clinical measurement, safety and clinical anaesthesia. The Royal College of Anaesthetists regulations allow an SHO to sit the Primary examination after twelve months of approved training, although eighteen months is recommended. Success in the Primary examination along with two satisfactory years of SHO anaesthesia training allow a trainee to apply for a SpR appointment and thus embark on a career as a specialist anaesthetist. In today's education jargon, the Primary examination is the summative assessment to complement the formative assessments carried out during the SHO years. In a sense, therefore, the Primary examination may be viewed as a screen for potential consultant anaesthetists in the future. An additional important point in the Royal College of Anaesthetists' regulations is that trainees are only allowed four attempts at each part of the FRCA. It is therefore essential that candidates for the examinations are well prepared and do not attempt the examinations until ready. How to prepare?

It is usually accepted that success in MCQs is primarily a test of core knowledge with a little technique related to understanding negative marking. Such core knowledge has to be acquired by regular reading of any of the standard large textbooks of anaesthesia, attendance at lectures and courses and perusal of the relevant specialist journals. Experience of the OSCEs from its introduction into the Part Three of the old FRCA indicated that clinical experience and practice in mock OSCEs were needed for success in this section of the examination. This leaves the Vivas. Clearly core knowledge is also needed for this type of examination as well as practice with mock events. However these may not be sufficient. The vivas consist of 'structured questions'. This means that all candidates at a particular viva session, in the interests of fairness and to avoid examiner bias, are asked the same questions. In addition, questions are reused, if they prove to be discriminating, at subsequent examinations. Inevitably a 'structured answer' begins to emerge for the successful questions. One might think that remembering questions might help subsequent examinees! However there is a large bank of questions and in addition many studies have shown that the way a candidate answers a viva question in front of the examiners is just as important as the actual knowledge. Nevertheless the concept of a structured way of considering viva questions is important. How is this to be done?

Mark Blunt and John Urquhart have brought together the disparate information needed to address the topics in Viva Two of the Primary FRCA. This book is not intended to be absolutely all encompassing – indeed such a work would probably be incomprehensible. It does however, lay out the topics in a logical order, and indicate the structures required for a candidate to answer the questions correctly. To be successful at a viva one needs to appear confident, but not *too* confident, listen carefully to the questions, speak up (the ambient noise level at viva sessions is often high and the examiners may have difficulty in hearing your answer), answer only what is asked and structure your answer in a logical order and be well prepared. The latter point is the most important, particularly in the light of the limited number of attempts now allowed at the FRCA. For the trainee, as part of your preparation for the Primary FRCA, this book and its companion volume (Urquhart JC and Blunt MC *The Anaesthesia Viva: Volume 1*) will give you the necessary starting position for the knowledge required to pass the examination.

Those of us engaged in busy consultant clinical practice or inhabiting the mythical 'ivory towers', for whom examinations are but a distant memory, might be forgiven for thinking a book such as this has little relevance to our day to day activities. However, regardless of where we practice there is always the potential embarrassment of the question we cannot answer. Indeed it is often the simplest ones which are most difficult. Study of this book will help to avoid such events and may well improve our clinical practice to the potential benefit of our patients.

Leo Strunin
BOC Professor of Anaesthesia
Director Anaesthetics Unit
Saint Bartholomew's and
The Royal London School of Medicine and Dentistry
Queen Mary's and West Field College
University of London

CONTENTS

2. QUESTIONS ON MEASUREMENT

3. QUESTIONS ON CLINICAL ANAESTHESIA

4. QUESTIONS ON ANATOMY

THE ANAESTHESIA VIVA
(PHYSICS, MEASUREMENT, CLINICAL ANAESTHESIA, ANATOMY, AND SAFETY)

Of all medical examinations the viva has caused the greatest fear amongst candidates. The Royal College has made determined efforts over the years to ensure the examiners are fair. This has been successful such that the well-prepared candidate can be reasonably sure of a fair 'hearing'. We hope that this series of books will help to increase the candidate's confidence and enable him or her to succeed in this part of the examination. We also believe that these books will be of value to teaching staff by offering a set of questions with researched answers on those subjects such as physics and measurement, that come less readily to mind.

The new structure of the examinations leading up to the Fellowship of the Royal College of Anaesthetists has extended the scope of the first examination to contain the majority of the subjects that were formally tested separately in the part I and part II examinations. Furthermore, the College has published a syllabus for the first time. This is absolutely vital reading for all candidates who may find that there are a number of subjects that are specifically mentioned that they were not expecting to be asked.

The viva examination offers candidates an unsurpassed opportunity to demonstrate both their knowledge and their ignorance. It is almost impossible to pass the viva without knowledge, however it is very much easier to pass with good technique. This is best learnt by repeated practice, something that can be done amongst candidates, with senior staff within the hospital or in formal examination courses.

The following points of technique are worth stressing. Although examiners try to be impartial it is important to look smart and interested when you arrive in the examination hall. Sit up, listen to the questions, sound confident and don't mumble. Take a little time before answering to order your thoughts, and ideally start with a broad overview of the answer. This should help you remember all the points you want to make and demonstrates an organised and logical mind. It also gives you more time to think! The examiner who has merely to guide the candidate in the direction he wishes to go is more likely to be impressed by the same knowledge than the one who has to wring each point out of the candidate.

This book starts the answer to many of the questions with a short sentence overview or with the most important point, and this is denoted by the highlighted text:

➡ **An overview gives you time to think and shows the examiner an organised and logical mind.**

The questions within the book are loosely divided into chapters according to the published description of the scope of the second Primary viva (Physics, Measurement, Safety and Clinical Anaesthesia). In addition there is a separate chapter on Anatomy. Candidates may want to retain the book for their Final examination work.

It should be remembered that candidates for the Primary are not expected to have done or seen everything. Similarly, candidates are not expected to know everything about all the anaesthetic equipment in use in the UK but they are expected to know all about the equipment that they use daily. Questions in the exam may start with an introductory question ("What vaporiser do you use in theatre?"). This allows the candidate to choose equipment that they are familiar with and therefore are reasonably expected to know their functions, advantages and dangers; they should also understand the principles underlying those functions. Obviously this is difficult to mimic in this format so some of the questions in the book may be rather more specific (such as "How does the 'Tec 5 vaporiser work?").

Finally, it must be noted that this book is not designed to be a definitive text for the Primary exam. It is a collection of questions derived from our own experience of the exam process, those of our colleagues, and questions that have been tested on candidates in hospitals that we have worked in and courses we have taught on. We hope that it will offer some pointers to help candidates for this exam succeed.

1 QUESTIONS ON PHYSICS

1. HOW DOES A 'ROTAMETER' WORK?

➡ **A 'Rotameter' is a variable-orifice flowmeter that allows a continuous indication of gas flow.**

A bobbin is supported by the gas flow within a conical glass tube. As the flow increases the bobbin rises so there is more space around the bobbin. Thus the bobbin is suspended with a variable orifice around it, and the size of the orifice depends on the gas flow. The pressure drop across the bobbin is constant and equal to the weight (mass × gravity) of the bobbin divided by the area of its bottom. The area of the ring around the bobbin increases as the bobbin rises, so as the flow increases the pressure remains constant.

The flow around the bobbin is a mixture of laminar and turbulent flow, due to the complex shape of the orifice. At low flows the area of the orifice is small, and it behaves like a thin tube, with the flow being more laminar, whereas higher up the area is larger relative to the length of the bobbin, and it behaves more like a short constriction in a tube, so the flow is more turbulent. As the flow depends on both viscosity and density of the gas the Rotameter is calibrated for the specific gas that it will measure.

In order for the Rotameter to be accurate it must be vertical to prevent the bobbin touching the sides of the tube and sticking. The bobbin has fins cut into its upper surface to make it spin, and so reduce the risk of sticking due to build up of static or dirt. There is also a conductive strip or coating on the inside of the tube to reduce the build-up of electrostatic charges.

•••••••••••••••••••••••••••••••

2. WHAT IS NATURAL (RESONANT) FREQUENCY AND MECHANICAL DAMPING?

> ➡ **Damping is the tendency of a system to resist the oscillations caused by a sudden change.**

Mechanical damping (as opposed to electrical damping) is mainly seen in clinical practice in direct intravascular pressure measurements. The system used consists of a column of liquid (normally dextrose, though in the case of pulmonary artery wedge pressure reading this is a column of blood then a column of dextrose), connected to a transducer. This allows changes in pressure to be detected by movement of the column of fluid that acts as a piston on the transducer that then records the movement either using a displacement or strain gauge. The resulting signal is amplified and displayed as a waveform and a digital readout.

If a sudden stepwise fall in pressure is applied to this system (e.g. after flushing the cannula) it acts in much the same way as a weight suspended on a spring and there is a tendency for oscillations to continue in the system. These oscillations occur at a consistent frequency known as the 'resonant frequency' or the 'undamped natural frequency'. Damping is a measure of the ability of the system to suppress these oscillations. In an underdamped system the oscillations continue for a long time. In an overdamped system changes occur slowly but with no overshoot . A system is said to be critically damped (D = 1.0) when there is a rapid fall in the pressure but over-shoot is just avoided.

If a waveform is applied at constant amplitude but gradually increasing frequency then as the frequency approaches the natural frequency the amplitude recorded is increased. Then as the frequency increases beyond the natural frequency the record-ed amplitude falls to zero. The natural frequency therefore adds inaccuracy to the system, and attempts are made to increase the natural frequency until it is higher than the operating frequency of the system. In the case of a direct arterial monitor this is about 20Hz. It is in fact very difficult to keep the natural frequency from imposing on the recorded frequencies in practice as this requires short, stiff-walled, wide catheters with no connections and no air bubbles. It is therefore important to keep the distortion to a minimum and this is the function of the damping incorporated in the system.

As noted above if the system is overdamped then it is slow to respond to changes, though it avoids overshoot. The slow response is not desirable in a clinical system as the waveform generated is flattened and has falsely low systolic and falsely high dias-tolic pressures (note though that the mean is correct). If the system is underdamped then there is overshoot and falsely high systolic and low diastolic (due to the artifac-tual increase in the amplitude of the high frequency part of the curve). In fact critical damping is normally too much for clinical applications and a better result is found when D = 0.64 (known as optimum damping).

Overdamping is frequently seen in clinical systems due to the elasticity of the walls of the tubing, the presence of air bubbles in the system or clots within the cannula and these should be avoided.

....

3. WHAT IS A VENTURI?

➡ **A Venturi is a colloquial expression for a device which uses the Venturi principle, which is an application of the Bernouilli effect.**

The Venturi principle is that a fluid will be entrained by the drop in pressure which results from the fluid (normally a gas) passing through a constriction, i.e. the Bernouilli effect. This is seen in nebulisers, oxygen masks, and in suction equipment remote from the central pipeline supply.

High air flow oxygen enrichment devices (HAFOE): These are a common application of the Venturi principle. (The Hudson and MC type masks are variable-performance devices, and therefore not the same as the HAFOE type). The design of the masks permit the delivery of predictable oxygen fractions according to the fresh gas flow delivered, due to the Venturi principle; in other words, the oxygen flow is entraining a known ratio of room air.

It is possible to establish the O_2 flow rate and the entrained air flow ratio for a device with the following equations:

$$100a \times 21b = 30 \times \text{required FiO}_2$$

$$a + b = 30$$

Where a — oxygen flow rate, b = entrained air flow rate, and the patient's peak inspiratory flow rate does not exceed 30 l/min.

The Venticaire HAFOE is a typical system, and observes a convention of colour coding for oxygen delivery.

Colour	Delivered FiO$_2$	Fresh gas flow (l/min)
Blue	24%	2
White	28%	4
Orange	31%	6
Yellow	35%	8
Red	40%	10
Green	60%	15

Giovanni Venturi was an Italian physicist, and died in 1822.

••••••••••••••••••••••••••••••••

4.   WHAT IS THE BERNOUILLI EFFECT?

➡ **The Bernoulli effect is that fluid passes faster through a constriction, gaining kinetic energy, but losing potential energy and so reducing pressure. In this way the total energy is preserved, in accordance with Newtonian Law. If the Bernoilli effect is used to entrain a second fluid, this is known as the Venturi principle.**

This is not the same as, but is frequently confused with, the Coanda effect. The Coanda effect is that a substance flowing in a tube is attracted to the walls, and is the basis of some ventilators.

Daniel Bernoilli was a Swiss mathematician who died in 1782.

••••••••••••••••••••••••••••••

5.   WHAT IS THE COANDA EFFECT?

When there is a constriction in a tube there is a fall in the pressure of the fluid flowing through it. This is the basis of a venturi, but when the stream then flows along a solid surface (eg the wall of a wide tube) entrainment cannot occur against the wall so the pressure at this point remains low, and the flow tends to stick to the wall, so if there are two outlets the fluid is not evenly divided, but tends to flow down one limb or the other. This may explain some of the maldistribution of gases in the alveoli, or instances of myocardial ischaemia when there appear to be patent coronary arteries. The Coanda effect can be used to allow the control of the flow of gas down one of two tubes, by using a small volume switching flow. Once the flow is established down one of the tubes the switching flow can be stopped and flow will continue down the appropriate tube. This is the basis of fluid logic, and can be used in ventilators to reduce the number of valves and moving parts.

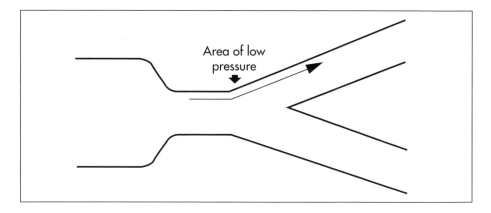

Area of low
pressure

••••••••••••••••••••••••••••••

6. WHAT IS THE DIFFERENCE BETWEEN A SOLID AND A FLUID?

➡ **A solid is compact and relatively dense. It maintains its shape unless subjected to large forces. Its molecules do not change position relative to one another and two adjacent solids will not mix. A fluid is a substance that will not sustain a shearing force.**

Liquids, gases and vapours are all fluids. A liquid is compact. Its molecules are constantly moving relative to one another, and because they are closely packed, collisions frequently occur. Because the molecules move freely, a liquid takes up the shape of the container in which it is confined, and its shape is affected by gravity. Different liquids in contact may or may not mix.

Gases and vapours are characterised as having no inherent boundary or volume; they expand to occupy the space in which they are confined. Different gases and vapours in contact will mix. Although the two terms are used synonymously, vapour is usually applied to the gaseous state at a temperature below the critical temperature for that substance (*see – **What do the following mean? – critical temperature***).

....

7. WHAT IS THE DIFFERENCE BETWEEN TEMPERATURE AND HEAT?

➡ **Temperature is a measure of the average kinetic energy of a substance; heat is energy.**

Temperature:

This is a measure of hotness and represents the average kinetic energy of a substance. Water at sea level and normal atmospheric pressure freezes at 0° Celsius and boils at 100°C. Absolute zero (0° Kelvin, K, or -273°C) is the point where all molecular motion ceases. Kelvin and Celsius are the same units of measurement, defined as 1/100th of the difference between the triple point (freezing point) of water (0°C) and the boiling point of water (100°C). However each describes a different scale; 0°K is absolute zero, whereas 0°C is the freezing point of water.

1 Cal = 1kcal = 1000 calories = 4200 joules.

Heat:

In order to raise the temperature (or average kinetic energy of the molecules) of a substance, heat must be added to it. One calorie raises the temperature of 1 gram of water from 14.5°C to 15.5°C. Latent heat of vaporisation is the heat required to vaporise a liquid; considerably more heat is required to vaporise a liquid than to raise its temperature from room temperature to boiling point. For water, the latent heat of vaporisation is 539 cal/g at 100°C. The latent heat of fusion is the heat required to melt a solid; for ice this is 80 cal/g at 0°C. Both these definitions are at atmospheric pressure.

....

8. WHAT DO THE FOLLOWING MEAN?

Critical temperature
Vapour and gas
Critical pressure
Critical flow

Critical temperature is defined as the temperature above which a substance cannot be liquefied by pressure alone.

A **vapour** is the term for a substance in the gaseous phase at or below its critical temperature. A **gas** applies to a substance that is above its critical temperature.

Critical pressure is the pressure required to liquefy a substance at its critical temperature.

Critical flow is the flow when the Reynold's number is 2000 and so the flow of the fluid is liable to change from laminar to turbulent.

$$\text{Reynold's number} = \frac{v\rho d}{\eta}$$

v linear velocity of the fluid
ρ density
d diameter of the tube
η viscosity

•••••••••••••••••••••••••••••••

9. IN WHAT WAY DOES THE OUTPUT FROM AN 'IDEAL' VAPORISER CHANGE AT HIGH ALTITUDE AND WHY?

➡ **In general vaporisers are designed to work by fully saturating a specific proportion of the gas flowing along the back bar.**

Therefore their output may be regarded as consisting of two separate volumes of gas; the first that has passed through the vaporiser chamber and contains anaesthetic vapour ideally at its saturated vapour pressure (svp); and the second consisting of the gas that contains no anaesthetic vapour that has by-passed the vaporising chamber.

As the svp of the vapour is unchanged at altitude the **partial pressure** of anaesthetic agent that comes out of the vaporising chamber will be unchanged. However the **concentration** of gas that leaves the chamber will be dependant on the ratio of that pressure to the total pressure (i.e. svp : P_{atm}). As the splitting ratio will be the same (it is this that the dial on the vaporiser changes), the concentration in the gas leaving the vaporiser will be changed inversely to the change in P_{atm}.

i.e. if:

P_{sea} = atmospheric pressure at sea level

P_{alt} = atmospheric pressure at altitude

C = concentration at sea level

C' = concentration at altitude

$$C' = C \times \frac{P_{sea}}{P_{alt}}$$

Therefore as the altitude increases and the barometric pressure falls the concentration from the vaporiser rises.

BUT the effect of the vapour does not depend on the concentration but on the partial pressure of the vapour. This has not changed, so the effect of using a vaporiser that is calibrated at sea level at the setting that one would normally use is the same. In fact in a normal vaporiser there are slight differences because the gas entering the vaporiser had a lower density so the resistance from the high-resistance pathway through the vaporising chamber will be slightly less. The vapour pressure in the chamber will therefore tend to approach svp more fully and so the partial pressure of vapour will be higher.

· ·

10. WHAT IS THE DIFFERENCE BETWEEN ABSOLUTE AND GAUGE PRESSURE?

➡ **Consider two tubes of mercury.**

Absolute pressure is most easily visualised as the height of a column of fluid which the pressure will support (though it should be noted that pressure is now strictly defined in terms of force per unit area). Absolute pressure is measured with respect to zero pressure (a vacuum). On the other hand gauge pressure is the pressure above or below atmospheric pressure. The two pressures may be visualised thus:

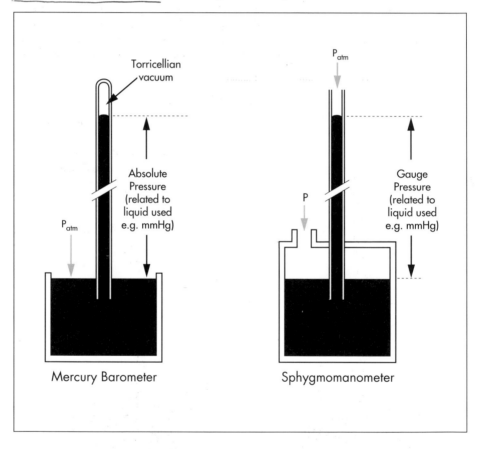

11. WHAT WOULD HAPPEN TO THE MENISCUS OF A MERCURY MANOMETER IF A FEW DROPS OF ISOFLURANE WERE INTRODUCED INTO THE VACUUM ABOVE IT?

➡ **This is a complicated sounding question that merely tests the understanding of some very simple physical principles – pressure and saturated vapour pressure.**

Atmospheric pressure (at sea level and room temperature) will support a column of mercury 760mm high in a liquid manometer. If a small amount of any liquid is introduced into the vacuum above there will be a pressure exerted on the top of the mercury column that is equal to the saturated vapour pressure of that vapour at room temperature. Thus the meniscus will fall so that the height of the column is equal to:

$$\text{Height} = P_{atm} - svp_{liquid}$$

Thus in our question:

$$\text{Height} = 760\text{mm} - 250\text{mm}$$
$$= 510\text{mm}$$

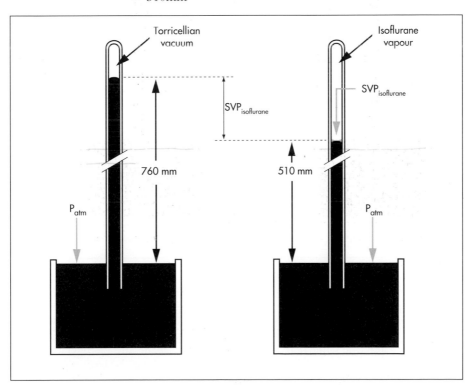

Note also that the answer to the question:

"What is present in the Torricellian vacuum?" is of course: Mercury vapour at svp_{Hg}.

••••••••••••••••••••••••••••••

12. WHAT IS 'FILLING RATIO' AND WHY SHOULD IT BE LESS THAN 1.0?

➡ **A cylinder containing gas can be easily filled to a set point by measuring the pressure in the cylinder. However one containing liquid needs another method to assess adequacy of filling and avoid overfilling.**

Because a cylinder of nitrous oxide contains liquid and has a pressure equal to the svp of nitrous oxide at the ambient temperature it is impossible to tell the amount of N_2O within the cylinder. This is in contrast to oxygen which remains as a compressed gas. In the latter case the amount of O_2 within the cylinder is equal to the absolute pressure of the cylinder contents in atmospheres × the volume of the cylinder. In order to measure the contents of a N_2O cylinder it is necessary to weigh the cylinder and subtract the mass of the empty cylinder. To equate this to a guide of the size of the cylinder and thus give an 'average density' of the contents this is divided by the mass of water the cylinder would hold:

$$\text{Filling Ratio} = \frac{\text{Mass of nitrous oxide in the cylinder}}{\text{Mass of water that the cylinder would hold}}$$

In our temperate climate the maximum permissible filling ratio is 0.75, though here as in tropical regions the most commonly used value is 0.67.

If we look at the pressure within a cylinder at various temperatures at the normal filling ratio of 0.67 and compare it with the pressure at a ratio of 0.77 where the cylinder at 20°C is almost totally full of liquid, the following can be seen:

Filling Ratio	Pressure at various temperatures (bar)		
	20°C	**40°C**	**60°C**
0.67	51	90	160
0.77	51	125	190

As can be seen the pressure at 40°C (above the critical temperature and hence with the cylinder containing only gas) has risen to 90 bar for the normal filling but is already approaching the pressure within an oxygen cylinder for the 'overfilled' cylinder. This is a temperature that is rare but does occur in the UK but is common in the tropics. However at 60°C the pressure of the normal cylinder has risen to 160 bar (approximately the same as a 'full' oxygen cylinder at the same temperature), but the 'overfilled' cylinder is at 190 bar and rapidly approaching the testing pressure of the cylinder, above which the cylinder may explode.

••••••••••••••••••••••••••••••••

13. HOW DOES A PRESSURE REGULATOR WORK?

➡ A diagram is invaluable in answering this question.

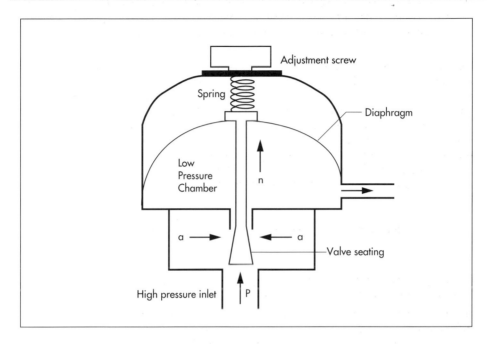

The low pressure chamber is enclosed on one side by the diaphragm. As gas enters under high pressure from the gas source, it passes through the valve seat and the pressure in the chamber beneath the diaphragm rises. This distends the chamber against the spring, and in so doing draws push rod upwards and the valve closed. The amount of gas delivered by the device is thus controlled by the position of the screw.

The push-rod is forced downwards by the combined action of the recoil of the diaphragm and the tension in the spring, S. This is opposed by the fresh gas flow and by the pressure in the low pressure chamber. The high pressure gas from source, P, acts on a cross-sectional area of the valve, a. The pressure in the chamber also deflects the push rod upwards, represented on the diagram as p.

$$S = Pa + pA$$

So, as the cylinder empties and P falls, the valve opens further to permit the same flow rate.

• •

14. WHAT HAPPENS TO THE PRESSURE WITHIN A NITROUS OXIDE CYLINDER AS IT IS DISCHARGED?

➡ **At room temperature nitrous oxide is below its critical temperature, and so the nitrous oxide cylinder contains both liquid and vapour under pressure, the pressure within the cylinder is therefore the saturated vapour pressure of N_2O at room temperature.**

The pressure is initially 52 bar, and the cylinder will remain at svp whilst there is still some liquid remaining within it, with liquid vaporising to maintain the pressure as vapour is released from the cylinder. Once the amount of N_2O within the cylinder has fallen to such an extent that all the liquid has vaporised the pressure within the cylinder falls as the vapour is released. Therefore it may be assumed that the pressure within the cylinder would fall thus:

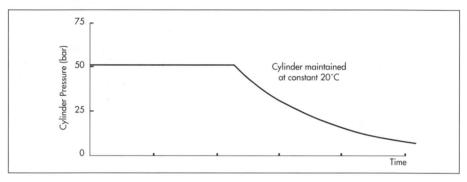

In fact this is not the case in practice because as the liquid vaporises it requires energy to overcome the latent heat of vaporisation, and this energy is supplied by heat from the N_2O itself, the cylinder and the surrounding air. Therefore the temperature of the liquid N_2O falls. This is why the outside of the cylinder is seen to condense water vapour and even to be covered with frost when the cylinder is in use. The pressure within the cylinder remains at the svp of N_2O. This falls with falling temperature so the pressure within the cylinder falls as the cylinder is continuously discharged. In fact if a 900l cylinder is discharged at 8 l/min it is impossible to see when the liquid is exhausted. However if the cylinder is switched off and allowed to return to room temperature whilst there is still liquid remaining then the pressure will return to 51 bar.

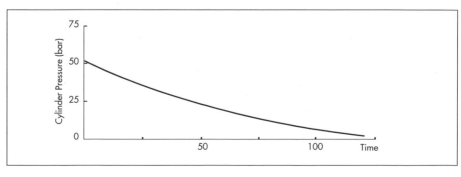

....

15. WHY CAN GASES BE USED FOR COLD CAUTERY ?

➡ **Cold cautery relies on the adiabatic expansion of gas as it leaves a capillary tube.**

Gas (normally either carbon dioxide or nitrous oxide) passes from a cylinder through a narrow capillary tube under pressure. As the gas leaves the capillary tube it expands and the pressure falls rapidly. As the gas cannot increase in volume fast enough to cope with the rapid fall in pressure part of the energy for this is supplied by a fall in temperature. An adiabatic change is one where the gas provides that thermal energy itself by a fall in temperature, rather than the energy coming from the surroundings.

Remember the combined ideal gas laws:

$$\frac{P_1 \cdot V_1}{T_1} = \frac{P_2 \cdot V_2}{T_2}$$

These show that for pressure to fall volume must increase or temperature fall, or in this case both must happen. The gas is now cold (temperatures of -70°C at the tip are normal) and it recovers that thermal energy from its surroundings. By directing the jet at the tissue in question cold cautery may be achieved.

•••••••••••••••••••••••••••••••

16. WHAT IS BOILING AND THE LATENT HEAT OF VAPORISATION?

Boiling is the process whereby a substance is converted from its liquid to its vapour phase. What happens is that bubbles of vapour form and then escape from the surface of the liquid. Obviously the pressure within the bubble is opposed by the pressure on the surface, that tends to stop the bubble escaping from the liquid. If the vapour pressure is equal to or greater than the pressure on the surface (i.e. the saturated vapour pressure is equal to or greater than the external pressure, commonly the atmospheric pressure) then the bubble is likely to escape and boiling occurs. The temperature at which the svp equals the ambient pressure is the temperature at which boiling occurs (by convention the 'boiling point' is the temperature at which the svp equals 1 atmosphere - 760 mmHg).

Latent heat of vaporisation is the energy required to fuel this process and convert a unit mass of liquid from the liquid phase to the vapour phase, at constant temperature and at specified pressure. At lower pressures (and therefore lower temperatures) the latent heat of vapourisation is larger.

•••••••••••••••••••••••••••••••

17. WHAT VENTILATOR DO YOU USE IN THEATRE?

➡ **Any ventilator will do; be ready to describe just one in detail. I recommend a Manley, because it is a classic of its type, because it is fairly simple to describe, and because all the examiners will know it.**

Roger Manley wrote up his ventilator in 1961, when Anæsthesia was still spelt with a diphthong and he was an SHO. His stated requirements for the ventilator were:

Minimal CVS effects;

It should provide as much information as possible, to compensate for the loss of the hand on the bag;

It should be small enough to stand on the anaesthetic machine;

It should operate from the fresh gas supply, with no ancillary power supply.

➡ **The key to the Manley is that it has two bellows.**

It also has two taps, and three valves. The minute volume is set on the flowmeters; it is therefore a minute volume divider. It is a volume-preset ventilator by the Hunter classification.

INSPIRATORY PHASE

The second bellows inflates the lungs due to the weight; the excursion of the second bellows is governed by a graduated scale, allowing for the tidal volume to be preset.

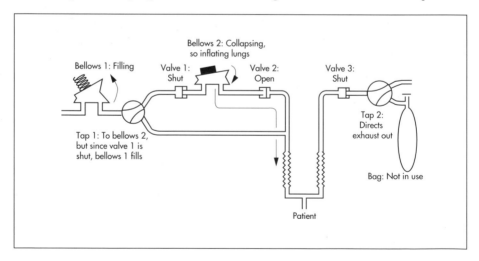

INSPIRATORY-EXPIRATORY CYCLING

Cycling depends entirely upon the opening of valve 1. This valve is opened by a lever mechanism when bellows 1 becomes full. This takes a variable period of time, dictated by the "duration of inspiration" dial. Valves 2 and 3 are operated by the changes in pressure in the system. It is therefore a volume-cycled ventilator.

EXPIRATORY PHASE

Valve 1 is open, allowing bellows 2 to fill. The patient's lungs are now open to the atmosphere via valve 3 and tap 2.

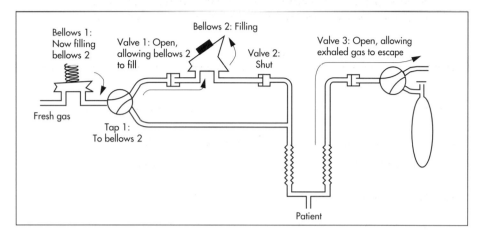

MANUAL VENTILATION

In this arrangement, the position of both taps is changed so that fresh gas is diverted to the patient, and the exhaust gas, instead of being allowed to escape, is diverted to the bag.

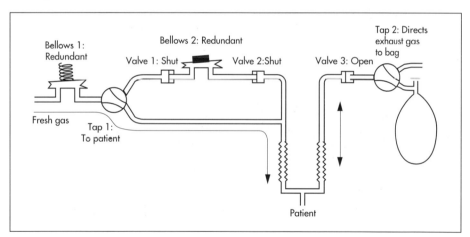

In manual mode, the ventilator is acting as a Mapleson D configuration; high gas flows are therefore required.

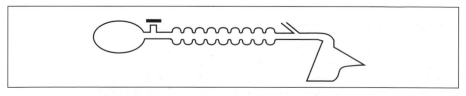

18. HOW DOES THE SUCTION WORK ON AN ANAESTHETIC MACHINE?

➡ **A suction device has four central components:**

- A pump or source of vacuum.
- A reservoir, containing an anti-foaming agent.
- A filter.
- A gauge, reading anticlockwise, with a yellow background.

➡ **Suction may be delivered by one of three methods:**

- By mechanical means; foot pump or hand-held device, both of which operate on a piston principle; these are used in field locations and for resuscitation.
- By venturi, employing a gas supply (usually oxygen); this is usually at locations where there is no central vacuum system, such as operating theatres in hospitals with no pipeline gases. Gases are from a cylinder supply, and suction is therefore driven by these gases. This is an expensive way of providing suction, as it consumes 20 l/min.
- By central vacuum supply, which is the commonest system in theatre and the one you should be ready to describe.

The source of suction is a pump (usually two) located centrally, which eliminates filtered gas to the atmosphere. This must be capable of sustaining a vacuum of not less than 400 mmHg below atmospheric. There will be a reservoir, which is protected by bacterial filters. The pipelines emerge from the wall alongside piped gas supplies at a Schrader valve, which is colour-coded yellow (in the UK) as is the pipeline within theatre. The standard for anaesthetic purposes is that it should take no more than 10 seconds to generate –500 mmHg, with a displacement capacity of 25 l/min. The tubing needs to have low resistance and low compliance.

The suction apparatus might deserve a diagram:

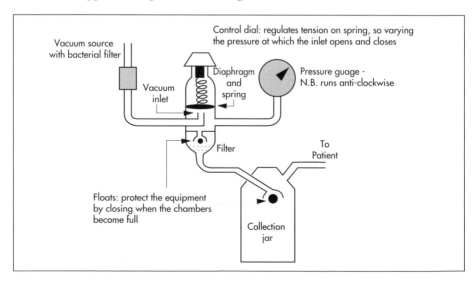

19. HOW CAN YOU ACCELERATE THE ADMINISTRATION OF INTRAVENOUS FLUID TO A PATIENT?

➡ **Start by describing the Hagen–Pouseille law:**

$$\text{Flow} = \frac{Pr^4\pi}{8\eta l}$$

Where P is the pressure across a tube, r is the radius, η the viscosity and l the length of tubing. The Hagen-Pouseille law applies to the intravenous cannula and also to the tubing connecting the cannula to the reservoir of fluid for administration. The important feature is that the radius of the tubing or cannula is applied to its fourth power, making this dimension the most relevant of all.

Using the Vialon *Insite* series, the flow rates are as follows:

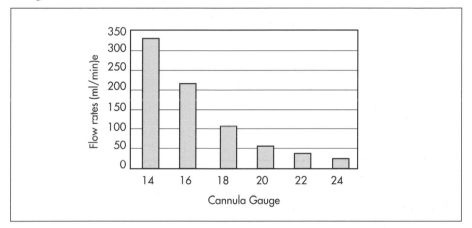

Hagen was a German engineer and Pouseille was a French physiologist.

The important feature, therefore, is to make sure that a cannula of appropriately-robust dimensions is inserted. Other means of accelerating flow include:

• Using short tubing, or accepting the reduction in flow caused by, for example, a blood warmer;

• Elevation of the fluid reservoir;

• Application of pressure to the fluid reservoir.

••••••••••••••••••••••••••••••

20. WHAT IS THE DIFFERENCE BETWEEN DIFFERENT TYPES OF DIATHERMY?

➡ Diathermy is the passage of an electrical current through tissue generating heat, in order to either coagulate blood vessels or cut through tissue, or both.

➡ The key expression when discussing diathermy is *current density*. With unipolar diathermy, when the current passes through the diathermy plate on the patient, there is a wide area exposed to the current and heating effect is minimal. At the forceps, however, the area exposed to the current and through which that current passes is very small, and the current density is therefore high; the heat generated is therefore considerable.

The current is of high frequency, 500 KHz - 1 MHz. (Mains supply is 50 Hz).

Cutting diathermy:

This uses current in an alternating sine-wave pattern.

Coagulation diathermy:

This uses current in a pulsed, sine wave pattern.

Unipolar diathermy:

The forceps represent one electrode, the plate on the patient the other.

Bipolar diathermy:

Current passes between the two blades of a forceps; no plate is required. This form is safer in the presence of a pacemaker. However only 40 Watts of energy can be delivered using bipolar diathermy, as opposed to 150 - 400 Watts with unipolar.

••••••••••••••••••••••••••••••

21. WHAT ARE THE PROBLEMS WITH DIATHERMY?

➡ **Injuries arising from the misuse of diathermy represent an ongoing source of litigation.**

The problems may be listed as follows:

Burns:

- Incorrect siting of the plate when using unipolar diathermy, with arcing and skin burns, because of increased current density.
- Ignition of skin preparation spirit – some types burn with an invisible flame.
- Inadvertent activation of diathermy while forceps are in contact with tissue remote from the operative site. This is why the forceps are kept in an insulated holder and a buzzer sound is used to indicate operation of the diathermy.
- Activation of the diathermy in contact with a metal object, which in turn is in contact with the patient and remote from the operative site.

Earthing:

In certain machines, the plate will be earthed. If this is so, and it is not properly applied, or if the connections to it are faulty, then current may go to earth by other routes. These include the ECG machine via the electrodes, and metal drip poles. Because current density at these sites is high, burns will result. Newer machines do not have earthed plates.

Pacemakers:

Unipolar diathermy may destabilise pacemakers, especially if the current traverses the chest.

Monitoring:

Activation of diathermy interferes with monitoring, especially with pulse oximetry and to a lesser extent with ECG.

....

22. WHAT DOES A TRANSDUCER DO?

➡ **An examiner of our acquaintance asks this question because the correct answer is rarely given.**

➡ **A transducer is quite simply a device which converts one form of energy into another, for the purposes of measurement. The second form of energy is normally electrical.**

A pressure transducer measures, indirectly, the pressure in the circulation, in a breathing system, or an infusion device. It consists of a semiconductor, whose shape is deformed by the action of the pressure in proportion to the pressure applied, altering its conductivity.

Flow transducers such as the Fleisch pneumotachograph deduce flow by measuring a pressure change. A small resistance to flow is imposed by a screen, thus creating a pressure difference between one side of the screen and another; this pressure difference is measured by a pressure transducer, and the flow deduced. A heater is included to prevent condensation of moisture and to ensure steady-state conditions within the device.

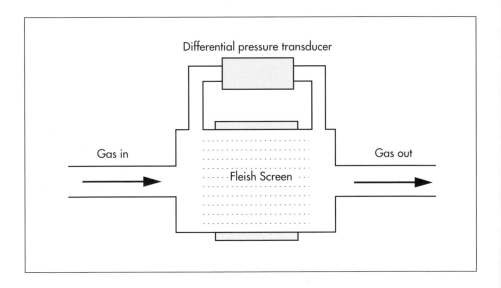

Differential pressure transducer

Gas in

Gas out

Fleish Screen

•••••••••••••••••••••••••••••••

23. WHAT IS A WHEATSTONE BRIDGE?

➡ **Many transducers used in medical practice depend on a physical change causing a change in their resistance. A Wheatstone bridge is a special arrangement of resistors designed to amplify this change in resistance.**

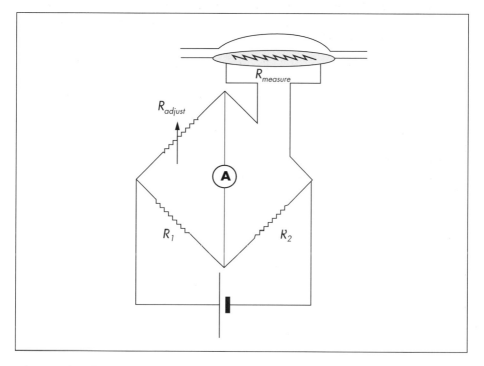

The simplest form of the Wheatstone bridge is designed so that it is balanced and there is no flow of current from one side to the other (i.e. the ammeter reads zero). This balance is achieved by adjusting the resistance in the adjustment leg to compensate for the change in the measurement leg. The resistance can then be calculated by:

$$\frac{R_{measure}}{R_{adjust}} = \frac{R_2}{R_1}$$

In practice however the current flow across the bridge is amplified and this is measured or displayed. Furthermore if **all** the resistances are part of the transducer (e.g. a strain gauge used to measure deflection of a diaphragm due to pressure) and these are set up so that two resistances increase whilst the other two decrease with the change in strain the electrical signal is amplified.

. . . .

24. WHAT IS A CAPACITOR GIVING AN EXAMPLE OF ITS IMPORTANCE IN PRACTICE?

➡ **A capacitor is a body that is able to hold electrical charge. It consists of two conductive plates separated by an insulator. Capacitance is a measure of that ability.**

The capacitor most frequently encountered in medical practice is the defibrillator. In this the capacitor is placed in a switched part of the circuit so it may be 'charged' by applying a voltage across the two plates and allowing the build up of charge. The voltage is considerably higher than mains voltage and this is achieved using a transformer. When the charging reaches a predetermined point the voltage is switched off but the charge in the capacitor remains. When the circuit is switched to 'defibrillate' this charge is released as a pulse of current (since current is merely charge per second), initially at the potential difference (i.e. voltage) that was present when the capacitor was charged. The circuit generally has an inductor to prolong the duration of the current flow. This duration is typically about 3 msec. The current flowing for that short time is in the order of 32 A initially at about 5000 V. this is enough to light over 2500 household light bulbs (but with them all going out one by one over the three microseconds duration of the pulse as the voltage falls to zero!). The energy supplied can be derived from the charge stored multiplied by the mean voltage (i.e. half the charging voltage).

The capacitor may be thought of as a rechargeable very high power battery with an ultra-short life.

....

25. WHAT IS IMPEDANCE AND WHEN IS IT OF VALUE IN MEDICAL MEASUREMENT?

➡ **Impedance is a measure of the obstruction to current flow through a capacitor.**

The resistance to current flow through a capacitor is not constant. When a d. c. circuit is switched on the current flowing through the capacitor rapidly falls to zero (by a exponential decline), and the potential difference (the voltage) across the capacitor rises. In an a. c. circuit the current is being continually switched on and off, and the capacitor does not reach steady state. The current flow through the capacitor follows the voltage change but is 90° out of phase.

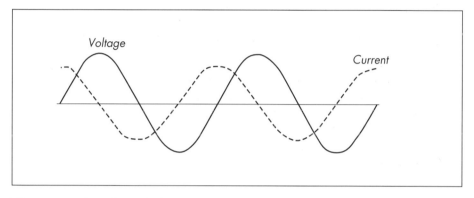

The current flow through the capacitor is proportional not to the voltage itself but to the rate of change of the voltage (dV/dt), and so is related to the frequency of the a. c. supply. As the current varies with frequency it is reasonable to assume that the hindrance to the current flow will change with frequency. This is termed the 'reactance' of the capacitor and it is inversely proportional to the frequency of the supply.

The circuit will also have a resistance (constant hindrance to flow that is not frequency dependant) and the resistance and the reactance are taken together to find the opposition to flow of the capacitance circuit. This is called the impedance and is quoted at a particular frequency.

All the tissues of the body can act as a capacitor and have an impedance. Furthermore this impedance is related to the constituents of that tissue, so if those constituents change then the impedance changes. Thus if the tissue between two electrodes contains increased blood (due to vasodilation) then the impedance will change. Another example is an increase in the air in the chest changes the thoracic impedance. Although the absolute value of the impedance is widely variable the change in value is relatively linear and the voltage **change** across the electrodes can be calibrated (in the latter case using expired spirometry for an initial calibration). This can be used as a rapid responding non-invasive measure of ventilation. Other uses include measurement of stroke volume in a beat-to-beat manner.

•••••••••••••••••••••••••••••••

26. WHAT ARE THE PRINCIPLE COMPONENTS OF A SCAVENGING SYSTEM?

➡ **A scavenging system is a group of components designed to transfer waste anaesthetic gases from the breathing system to a safe remote location.**

All scavenging systems consist of:

- A collecting device; a shroud around the exhaust valve, or a canopy over a recovering patient, although the latter is a rarity;
- A means of taking the gases away, by tubing. Scavenging connections are 30 mm diameter, to prevent inadvertent connection to the breathing system;
- A receiving system, in other words a reservoir of some description. A pressure relief valve is usual to prevent the possibility of barotrauma.
- An exhaust system to discharge the gases safely.

Passage of gases through the systems may be powered either by the patients expiration (passive systems) or by active means.

Passive scavenging:

This may be a simple tube leading out to atmosphere. The Cardiff Aldasorber is a canister of activated charcoal connected to the exhaust tubing, and extracts volatile anaesthetic agents but not N_2O. It weighs 1 kg when new and this allows calculation of the extent of its use and of the time to replace it.

Active scavenging:

This is able to cope better with the variation in gas flow rates that are seem in normal anaesthetic practice, and normally consists of a type of fan system that produces a constant low suction pressure (sub-anaesthetic pressure). Pipeline suction is inappropriate because a low-pressure system is needed for safety reasons. The source should remove 75 l/min. Other methods of driving scavenging systems include venturi systems.

The gases are collected and then ducted to a collecting system that must contain some form of reservoir, either a reservoir bag or an open-ended vessel. If this is a closed vessel then there should be a high pressure valve (10 cmH_2O) to avoid back-flow of gases if the capacity is exceeded or there is a blockage. It also needs a low-pressure valve (-0.5 cmH_2O) to allow air in when the expired gas flow does not meet the disposal system demands. These are unnecessary if the open vessel is used, as this effectively provides them via the opening. The air-break (as seen in the Ohmeda Active Gas Scavenging System) provides this:

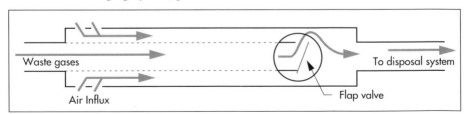

The exhaust system should then discharge the gases outside at a suitable site away from areas where personnel are working.

••••••••••••••••••••••••••••••••

27. WHY USE SCAVENGING?

➡ **Scavenging is the removal of waste gases from expired gases; it may be active or passive.**

In the 1970's concern about the risks of anaesthetic agents was highlighted by a number of studies looking at the effect of long-term exposure to trace levels of anaesthetic agents. Although the results are disputed there have been various claims of deleterious effects on the health of theatre personnel. Commonly quoted effects relate to pregnancy and include an increased risk of miscarriage in anaesthetists, the wives of anaesthetists and anaesthetic nurses and an increased incidence of female children to male anaesthetists. Illness amongst exposed staff is less well defined but may include an increased incidence of blood cell tumours (lymphoma and leukaemia) in female anaesthetists, however viral hepatitis is a much more common cause of occupational illness in anaesthetists.

There are also many reports of subjective symptoms such as fatigue, malaise and headaches. One only has to remember what one feels like after a paediatric list where high concentrations of volatile agents are used and scavenging is often less effective to realise this.

In 1989 the government introduced a code of practice called the 'Control of Substances Hazardous to Health' (COSHH). This is seen as the guidelines for implementation of the Health and Safety at Work Act (1974), and as such is a code that all employers (and hospitals) should follow. Scavenging is seen as a method of reducing the risk of exposure to potentially hazardous material, and as such it is the legal as well as moral responsibility of the anaesthetist to use scavenging to minimise the risks of exposure to both himself (or herself) and to other theatre personnel.

COSHH sets requirements for alternatives to mask anaesthesia, requires a named manager with responsibility for implementation of the regulations, a system of closed filling for vaporisers to be carried out in a fume cupboard, and minimum rates of air supply:

- Operating Theatres: $0.65 \text{ m}^3/\text{s}$
- Anaesthetic rooms: $0.15 \text{ m}^3/\text{s}$
- Prep rooms: $0.1 \text{ m}^3/\text{s}$
- Recovery: 15 air changes per hour.

It also lays down time weighted average exposure levels for volatiles, to be monitored by the use of personal samplers to be carried within the breathing area of the practitioner. These are:

- N_2O: 100 ppm (USA: 25 ppm)
- Isoflurane: 50 ppm (USA, for all volatiles, limit is 2 ppm)
- Enflurane: 20 ppm
- Halothane: 10 ppm

It became a criminal offence not to apply this act after the lifting of Crown Immunity.

•••••••••••••••••••••••••••••••

28. WHAT IS MICROSHOCK AND HOW IS IT PREVENTED?

➡ **The risk of ventricular fibrillation relates to the current density in the heart so a very small voltage within the heart can be just as lethal as a larger one applied to the skin of a hand.**

It is well known that the passage of an electrical current through the heart may lead to ventricular fibrillation. If the electrical current comes from touching a live wire with a hand and the current passes to earth via the feet most of that current passes through the non-cardiac tissues of the trunk, with only a small proportion passing through the heart. Thus a relatively large current is required to cause ventricular fibrillation. However if the current comes from an intracardiac catheter then almost all of the current will pass through the heart. In this case only a very small current is required to cause ventricular fibrillation (in the order of 150 μA). It should also be noted that as the current density is increased the voltage similarly can be reduced so it is possible to get microshock with battery voltages (12 V) or less.

The main cause of current reaching the heart is 'leakage' currents. These are the currents that flow other than in the designed direction, such as to the equipment casing. For these leakage currents to be dangerous they must be large enough to cause ventricular fibrillation and must reach the heart. Equipment that is intended for use in direct contact with the heart must meet BS5724 type CF. This must have a maximum leakage current of under 50 μA even if there is a 'single fault' and also must have a 'floating' circuit. Furthermore in the case of equipment connected to the patient by intravenous cannulae the risk of shock is said to be reduced by using low-ionic liquid in the system (i.e. 5% dextrose rather than normal saline).

....

29. WHICH PRODUCES A HIGHER PRESSURE - A 2 ML OR A 20 ML SYRINGE?

➡ **The pressure of the injecting liquid is dependant on the force exerted on the syringe and the area over which that force acts.**

Assuming the same force is applied. This question asks for knowledge of a very fundamental principle.

$$P = \frac{f}{a}$$

P = pressure developed

f = force of injection

a = cross-sectional area

The smaller the cross-sectional area the higher the pressure developed, and the answer to the question is that the 2 ml syringe allows the higher pressure to be developed.

....

30. WHY SHOULD YOU NOT INJECT INTO A CANNULA PLACED IN THE ANTE-CUBITAL FOSSA WHEN PERFORMING INTRAVENOUS REGIONAL ANAESTHESIA ?

➡ **It is easy to develop very high pressures with a syringe, and so cause extravasation of injectate or to overcome the pressure of the occluding cuff during IVRA.**

It is easily possible to develop forces of 25-50 N by pressing on a syringe plunger (this is the equivalent of 2.5-5 kg-weight). The internal diameter of the 2 ml syringe is 8 mm which gives a cross-section (π x radius^2) of 0.00005 m^2. Thus the pressure developed is 500-1000 kPa which is 30-60 times systolic pressure (120 mmHg), and 15 to 30 times the usual cuff pressure (250 mmHg). Even a 20 ml syringe with an internal diameter of 18 mm will allow the development of pressures of 100-200 kPa (3 to 6 times the cuff pressure). Thus it is important to allow the compliance of the venous system, and the resistance to flow of a small-bore cannula a chance to absorb the pressure before the cuff is reached. The best way to do this is to place a small cannula in a small vein in the back of the hand and inject slowly.

•••••••••••••••••••••••••••••••••

31. WHAT IS HIGH-FREQUENCY VENTILATION?

➡ **High frequency ventilation is defined as ventilation at more than four times the normal rate, and requires much smaller tidal volumes (1 - 3 ml/kg) than conventional ventilation.**

High frequency positive pressure ventilation (HFPPV) is fast IPPV, at 60 - 120 cycles per minute (cpm), via a conventional tracheal tube. *High frequency oscillation* (HFO) depends on a sinusoidal pattern of flow generated by a loudspeaker cone. The Hayak oscillator requires no tube, but uses a cuirass. *High frequency jet ventilation* (HFJV) is the commonest HFV mode.

High frequency jet ventilation

The equipment consists of the following:

1. High frequency jet ventilator.

2. Mixer unit.

3. O_2 and air sources (both at 4 bar).

4. Portex gas monitoring tracheal tube or Mallinkrodt "Hi-Lo" tube. Some such tubes have two additional lumens, one each for the jet and for sampling.

High frequency ventilation can be used in thoracic and laryngeal surgery, and in ITU; in acute respiratory distress syndrome and when withdrawing ventilation, the patient can talk and breathe. In thoracic surgery, it is of great help in the management of bronchopleural fistula. A form of HFJV takes place at bronchoscopy, with the Sanders injector.

•••••••••••••••••••••••••••••••••

32. WHAT ARE THE BASIC SI UNITS?

➡ **The *Système Internationale* units were introduced by the General Conference on Weights and Measures in 1960 and are based on the Metric system. There are base units and derived units.**

Base units:

Unit	Unit of:	Definition:
Metre	Length	The distance occupied by 1,650,763.73 wave-lengths of light from gaseous krypton. The original bar of platinum-iridium against which the metre was calibrated ceased to be used after concerns about its consistent length over time.
Second	Time	The definition relates to the frequency of radiation emitted by Caesium-133. It is also roughly $\dfrac{1}{24 \times 60 \times 60}$ of the time taken for the earth to complete one revolution.
Kilogram	Mass	There is a standard cylinder of platinum-iridium against which the kilogram is calibrated. It is about 37 mm in each dimension and is kept near Paris.
Ampere	Electric current	The current in two straight parallel wires 1 metre apart in a vacuum which will produce a force of 2×10^7 newtons/metre on each of the wires.
Kelvin	Temperature	$0°K$ is $-273.16°C$. The exact definition is, $1K = 1/273.16$ of the thermodynamic scale temperature of the triple point of water, where water in solid, liquid and gaseous state are in equilibrium.
Candela	Luminous intensity	Involves the intensity of a body at the freezing point of platinum.
Mole	Substance	The quantity of a substance containing Avogadro's number of particles (6.022×10^{23}), the number of particles as atoms in 12 grams of ^{12}Carbon.

Derived units:

Unit	Unit of:	Definition:
Newton	Force	Force = mass x acceleration. 1 Newton = the force required to accelerate a mass of 1 kg by 1 m/s^2.
Pascal	Pressure	Pressure = force/area. 1 Pascal = 1 N/m^2.
Joule	Energy, work	Potential energy is the energy possessed by a body because of its position; kinetic energy is the energy of a body due to its motion. 1 Joule is the work done (energy used) when a force of 1 N moves 1 metre.
Watt	Power	Power is the rate of doing work, = work/time. 1 Watt = 1 joule/second.
Hertz	Frequency	1 Hertz = 1 cycle/second.

As a postscript, here are Newton's Laws of Motion:

1. A body continues in its state of rest or in its uniform motion in a straight line unless acted upon by an external force.

2. When a force acts on a body, the rate of change of momentum in the body is proportional to the force and is in the same direction as that in which the force acts.

3. For every action there is an equal and opposite reaction.

The law of conservation of energy is that energy can be neither created nor destroyed, but only transformed from one state to another.

• •

33. HOW DOES A LASER WORK?

➡ **LASER is an acronym of Light Amplification by Simulated Emission of Radiation.**

It produces an intense beam of light that is monochromatic (of one wavelength). The beam is emitted as a parallel stream of photons with little or no divergence so it can be used to deliver a large amount of energy accurately to small areas of tissue.

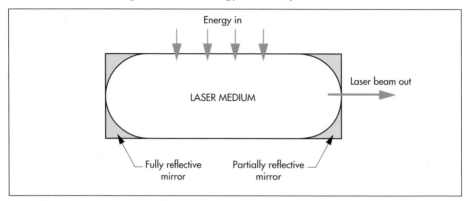

The laser works by absorbing energy from an external source (e.g. a flashlight or high-voltage discharge). This energy may then be released as a photon of a specific wavelength. If this is then reflected back into the laser medium and meets another excited atom, that atom releases its energy in the form of another photon that is parallel and in phase with the other photon. These may then cause a further similar reaction, and the resulting chain-reaction leads to release of an intense form of light in phase and parallel. This is emitted from the lazing chamber and in most medical cases is directed onto the target tissue by a fibre-optic wand.

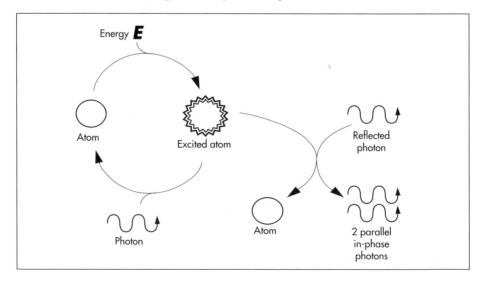

· ·

34. WHY ARE DIFFERENT LASERS USED THERAPEUTICALLY AND WHAT ARE THE GENERAL AND SPECIFIC RISKS THAT RELATE TO THE ANAESTHETIST?

➡ **The most common lasers in therapeutic use are carbon dioxide, argon and Nd:YAG (neodymium : yttrium–aluminium garnet).**

The differing mediums are used in order to vary the depth of penetration, the wavelength of the light and the power of the beam.

- *Carbon dioxide* light is infra-red and is absorbed by water that is vaporised, destroying the tissue contents. Thus these lasers are used as a scalpel to cut into tissues with haemostasis.
- *Argon* lasers produce light in the blue-green area of the visible spectrum and so are maximally absorbed by red tissues. Thus it tends to be used directed at the small vessels within the transparent tissue of the eye.
- The *Nd:YAG* laser is a near infra-red laser that is used for penetrating deeply into tissues.

The **general dangers** of laser usage are due to the non-divergent beam that therefore has almost no loss of power as the distance from the source is increased. The greatest danger is of light entering the eye where it will tend to burn the retina as well as damaging the aqueous and vitreous humours, cornea and lens. Indeed the major danger is of light landing on the 'blind spot' and damaging the optic nerve as this can cause irreversible total blindness. Surfaces around the target tissue should be non-reflective as the dangers are compounded by reflection in glossy surfaces. The lesser danger is of damage to skin or tissues distant to the target tissue.

The specific dangers for anaesthetists relate to the risk of fire in the oxygen-enriched atmosphere in and around the airway. This is most commonly encountered in ENT procedures, but it should be remembered that surgical drapes can hold a high concentration of oxygen or combustion-supporting nitrous oxide that can be ignited if the laser is accidentally directed below them.

The following measures should be taken to reduce the risks:

- Flammable anaesthetic agents should not be used (including nitrous oxide).
- Laser-resistant endotracheal tubes should be used. A standard tube is highly flammable in the airway environment and will ignite if the laser beam is directed at it, and the technique of covering this with silver-foil may cause damage to the larynx or the vocal cords and may not shield the tube fully. It should however be noted that even laser-resistant disposable tubes will not withstand direct laser light for any length of time.
- Inspired oxygen should be diluted with air, ideally to an F_IO_2 of 0.25 or less, if the patient can cope with this.
- Black-coloured instruments reduce the risk of reflections.
- Damage to near-by tissues should be avoided by covering them with wet swabs.

•••••••••••••••••••••••••••••••

35. HOW DO YOU MONITOR HFJV?
WHAT ARE THE ADVANTAGES AND
DISADVANTAGES OF THE TECHNIQUE?

➡ **If the examiner asks this, you will be doing very well.**

Monitoring HFJV:

- By arterial blood gas analysis. This is the best method, but cannot provide continuous data.
- Single-breath end-tidal CO_2 using a capnograph and the machine in manual mode.

Advantages of HFJV:

1. There is increased cardiovascular stability compared with conventional IPPV.
2. There is less barotrauma, which is of benefit to both the lung and any surgical anastomosis.
3. The surgeons say that there is a better operative field.
4. Double lumen tube is not required.
5. It is possible to operate on a pulmonary lobe without letting down the lung. In severe pulmonary disease, the shunt imposed by deflation of a lung can be severe and limits the duration the lung can be deflated.

Disadvantages of HFJV:

1. Heat loss – the inspired gas can be warmed, but the entrained gas cannot.
2. Moisture loss – however a humidifier can be attached via a T-piece at the ventilator, delivering 20 ml/hr of saline.
3. It is impossible to use a volatile agent, so the technique requires the technique of total intravenous anaesthesia.

••••••••••••••••••••••••••••••

2 QUESTIONS ON MEASUREMENT

1. WHAT IS THE MINIMUM MONITORING THAT YOU CONSIDER APPROPRIATE FOR A DAYCASE D & C?

➡ **The most indisputable level of monitoring for ANY case is the continued presence of an anaesthetist, and this should be stated first.**

Exactly what monitoring is used above and beyond this will vary from anaesthetist to anaesthetist, however an answer may be reasonably based on the recommendations of the Association of Anaesthetists (*Recommendations for Standards of Monitoring during Anaesthesia and Recovery*, Revised Edition 1994, pub: The Association of Anaesthetists of Great Britain and Ireland).

Monitoring should commence before induction and be continued until recovery is complete.

What monitoring should be used can then be divided into two;

Monitoring the Anaesthetic Machine

- The anaesthetic machine must have been checked before use.
- The oxygen supply should be monitored by a device which has an audible alarm measuring the concentration actually delivered to the patient.
- The breathing system should be monitored by watching the movement of the reservoir bag, which should help detect leaks, disconnection or excessive pressure.
- This should be supplemented by capnography.

Monitoring the Patient

- Clinical observations should include:
  colour of mucosal membranes
  response to surgical stimulus
  movements of chest wall and reservoir bag
  palpation of pulse
  auscultation of breath sounds.
- A continuous display of heart rate, pulse volume (i.e. plethysmography) and oxygen saturation (this is normally available from the pulse oximeter).
- A continuous display of ECG.
- Non-invasive blood pressure should be taken and recorded regularly.

••••••••••••••••••••••••••••••

2. WHAT IS THE MOST ACCURATE MEASUREMENT ON THE DINAMAP?

➡ **The most accurate measurement is the mean pressure. You would now be asked to explain why.**

Mean arterial pressure was the only measurement taken by the early machines. The name of the machine created by Datascope was derived from "**D**evice for **I**ndirect **N**oninvasive **A**utomated **M**ean **A**rterial **P**ressure" which emphasises the point.

The Dinamap inflates the cuff to 180 mmHg, and then deflates. In subsequent measurements it will inflate the cuff to 50 mmHg above the previous systolic reading (if it has not been turned off in the meantime, in which case it reverts to the default setting). Thereafter it deflates, with the amplitude of the pulsation being recorded as an electrical signal through the action of a transducer. The pressure will slowly increase, reach a maximum, and then decrease as the cuff goes down. The systolic is taken as the first pressure peak.

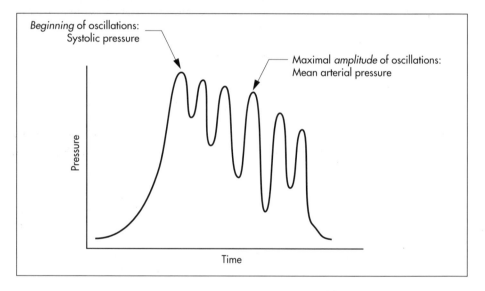

The mean arterial pressure is taken as the lowest pressure at which pulsations are maximal. The cuff deflates to five steps below the disappearance of the pulse; the disappearance is taken as diastolic, but is the least accurate of the measurements.

The machine uses a 8080 8-bit microprocessor; a modern PC will be based on at least a 80486 microprocessor and use 32-bit technology. The cuff serves two purposes, occluding the arterial pulsation as well as measuring wave amplitude.

$$\text{Mean arterial pressure} \quad = \frac{(2 \times diastolic) + systolic}{3} \quad \text{or}$$

$$diastolic + \frac{(systolic - diastolic)}{3}$$

••••••••••••••••••••••••••••••

3. WHAT IS THE FICK PRINCIPLE?

➡ **The Fick principle is a method of calculating blood fl⸱ organ by measuring the rate of loss (or uptake) of a sub⸱⸱⸱ change in its concentration as it passes through the organ.**

Classically the Fick principle was used to calculate cardiac output by measuring the venous and arterial oxygen concentration and the rate of uptake of oxygen by the lungs. This technique used a Benedict Roth spirometer and a soda-lime canister, allowing measurement of the change of volume to equate to the oxygen uptake.

The formula is then used thus:

$$\text{Cardiac output} = \frac{\text{Uptake } O_2}{(\text{arterial} - \text{venous}) \, O_2 \text{ Concentration}}$$

The Fick principle has been used frequently to measure the blood supply to many organs, either using oxygen, carbon dioxide or another endogenous substance or by using exogenous substances (such as indocyanine green).

•••••••••••••••••••••••••••••••

4. HOW DOES A pH ELECTRODE WORK?

➡ **The pH electrode is an ion-selective electrode that relies on the electricity generated by the movement of H^+ ions between the sample liquid and a reference buffer at known $[H^+]$.**

The sample and the buffer are separated by hydrogen-ion sensitive glass so the development of current depends on the movement of hydrogen ions alone. The buffer is then in contact with a Ag/AgCl electrode and there needs to be a reference electrode in contact with the blood. This electrode is separated from the blood by a semi-permeable membrane to avoid protein contamination and the electrode is kept in contact with the blood by a saturated potassium chloride solution.

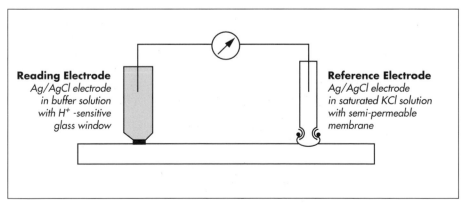

Reading Electrode
*Ag/AgCl electrode
in buffer solution
with H^+ -sensitive
glass window*

Reference Electrode
*Ag/AgCl electrode
in saturated KCl solution
with semi-permeable
membrane*

•••••••••••••••••••••••••••••••

. WHAT DOES pH MEAN?

pH is a measure of the hydrogen ion concentration in a liquid. It is the negative logarithm (base 10) of the hydrogen ion concentration [H$^+$].

The normal pH of water is 7 and this is said to be neutral pH as in water the [H$^+$] is equal to the [OH$^-$]. It should be noted that the pH scale is a logarithmic one and therefore each fall in pH of one unit is equal to a tenfold increase in the hydrogen ion concentration (pH of 8 is 10 nmol[H$^+$]/l and pH of 7 is 100 nmol[H$^+$]/l). Normal body pH of 7.4 equates to 40 nmol[H$^+$]/l.

Although the scale is not linear it is actually fairly close to linear over the middle of the range normally experienced in clinical practice.

· ·

6. HOW CAN YOU TURN A pH ELECTRODE INTO A CO₂ ELECTRODE?

➡ **The Severinghaus electrode that is used to measure CO₂ in most blood-gas machines is a modified pH electrode.**

The reading electrode with its buffer solution behind a H$^+$-sensitive glass window is retained intact. It is encased in another container filled with a bicarbonate solution that acts as the reference (and also contains the reference Ag/AgCl electrode). This solution is covered with a plastic membrane that is gas-permeable and separates the bicarbonate solution from the blood sample itself. As the membrane is gas-permeable it allows the carbon dioxide in the bicarbonate solution to reach equilibrium with the blood. The pH within the bicarbonate solution is then dependent on the Henderson-Hasselbalch equation. The pH change due to the addition of carbon dioxide is measured by the pH electrode.

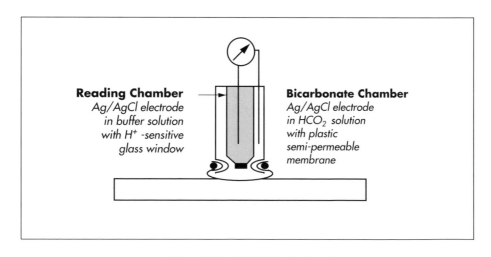

Reading Chamber
*Ag/AgCl electrode
in buffer solution
with H$^+$ -sensitive
glass window*

Bicarbonate Chamber
*Ag/AgCl electrode
in HCO₂ solution
with plastic
semi-permeable
membrane*

· ·

7. WHAT ARE THE SOURCES OF ELECTRICAL INTERFERENCE IN BIOLOGICAL SIGNALS?

➡ **Electrical interference is either due to external causes or to the patient. The former is most commonly due to the a. c. mains current, and the latter due to skeletal muscle action potentials either due to movement or shivering.**

Mains current interference may occur if there is capacitive coupling between the mains and the patient. If a live conductor is close to the patient (though not touching) then that lead tends to act as one plate of a capacitor, with the patient as the other plate. The circuit is completed as both are connected to earth. As the current in the live lead alternates between positive and negative the charge on the other side of the capacitor alternates similarly. This can be picked up on recording electrodes (e.g. the ECG) and is seen as a 50 Hz signal on the recording. This can be reduced either by moving the patient away from the live conductor, or by providing an earthed screen between the two 'plates' of the capacitor. This then discharges the charge from the live plate to earth and reduces the effect. Screened electrode leads consist of a wire mesh around the electrode that is connected to earth. A further cause of mains interference is by the interaction between the patient as a conductor in the changing magnetic field generated by the electromagnetic effect of the live conductor.

The most effective way to remove these signals is to have a 'common' lead in the ECG equipment that allows subtraction of those parts of the signal that are common to all the electrodes - called common mode rejection.

Patient interference is due to the presence of other electrical activity that is being measured. Anything that increases the amplitude of these signals, or reduces the amplitude of the signal being measured will increase the effect of this interference. As noted above the most common problem is due to skeletal muscle activity especially during shivering, and everything should be done to ensure that the measured signal is maximised (by reducing the resistance at the patient connection) and that activity is minimised by keeping the patient warm and asking them to stop moving.

••••••••••••••••••••••••••••••

8. WHAT METHODS ARE AVAILABLE TO MEASURE CO_2 IN GASES?

➡ **The method seen most frequently in anaesthetic practice uses absorption of infrared light.**

For measurement methods to be of use to anaesthetists they must be:

- accurate to clinical levels
- repeatable
- be easy and relatively quick to calibrate, and allow quick re-calibration if there is drift in the calibration
- have a short response time so breath-to-breath measurements can be taken and the shape of the waveform displayed
- small enough to fit into the monitoring 'stack'
- ideally they should measure other respiratory gases of interest particularly inhalational anaesthetic agent levels
- the readings should not be significantly affected by the presence of other gases or water vapour

There are two methods seen in anaesthetic practice and other methods that may be of value in a research setting or in specific situations.

Practical methods that are seen in theatre use

- **Infrared absorption**

   A gas will absorb infra-red (IR) radiation (wavelength 1 - 40 μm), causing it to vibrate if it consists of more than one atom, and if those atoms are of different elements; so CO_2 N_2O, H_2O and volatile agents will absorb IR, while O_2 will not. The IR wavelength absorbed depends on the species (maximal at 4.26 μm for CO_2), and this allows IR absorption to identify different gases, the amount of light absorbed being in proportion to the amount of gas present. If the absorption at specific wavelengths is then compared with that of a reference gas the concentration of carbon dioxide (and in some cases other gases) may be measured. Modern infrared analysers display concentrations of many respiratory gases (including carbon dioxide, nitrous oxide and volatile anaesthetic agents). However errors may be seen due to interference by oxygen broadening the carbon dioxide spectra, and interference between gases (especially nitrous oxide and carbon dioxide as the spectra overlap substantially), also water vapour absorbs infrared light and this can cause falsely high readings. If the radiation is pulsed, sound is generated in proportion to the amount of gas present; this is the photoacoustic variation of spectroscopy, popular in Denmark but not the UK.

- **Raman scattering**

   Gas is drawn from the breathing system and is exposed to monochromatic light from an argon laser. The energy from the light is absorbed by the intermolecular bonds and then is partial re-emitted at new wavelengths by the molecules. The wavelength shift and the scattering may be used to measure the concentration of the gases in the system. Thus the technique allows measurement of all the gases normally of interest in a breathing system (including carbon dioxide, nitrous oxide, oxygen, nitrogen and volatile anaesthetic agents). It is small and portable, and the gases may be returned to the breathing system unchanged, however it does not have the response rate suitable for paediatric monitoring with small tidal volumes and high respiratory rates.

Other Methods

- **Mass Spectrometer**

    Gas is drawn from the breathing system into the spectrometer where it is ionised then exposed to a magnetic field in a vacuum chamber. The various gases are separated according to their mass : charge ratio. The concentration of various gases of known mass : charge ratio may then be calculated. The spectrometer is highly accurate, reproducible and allows the measurement of many gases, however it is very bulky and expensive, and is susceptible to damage from water and some drugs. The gases cannot be returned to the breathing system so should be scavenged.

- **Calorimetric measurement**

    If carbon dioxide is hydrated the result is carbonic acid which can therefore be measured by pH-sensitive means (e.g. using colour change). The FEF detector uses this principle and is very small and portable. It does however only give a crude assessment of CO_2 level (low, normal, high) but is useful in resuscitation to confirm the presence or otherwise of exhaled carbon dioxide.

• •

9. WHAT IS A CAPNOGRAPH?

➡ **The capnograph is regarded by many as the single most useful monitor in theatre.**

A capnograph is a device which records and displays the CO_2 concentration. It produces a capnogram, which is a graphical plot of CO_2 against time. A capnometer is an instrument for measuring the numerical concentration of CO_2. Thus, all capnographs are capnometers, but a capnometer need not display a capnogram.

A realtime capnogram waveform displays a trace at 12.5 mm/sec, demonstrating fine detail and sudden changes in morphology. A trend capnogram waveform displays at 25 mm/min, demonstrating gradual changes over time. The delay time is the sum of the transit time and the rise time, where the transit time is the time taken for a sample to be delivered from the point of interest to the analyser, and the rise time is the time taken by the capnographic cell to register from 10% to 90% of a step change after the sample has entered the measuring chamber. The latter is also known as the response time, and is important as it must be less than the time taken for one breath.

There are two common structural arrangements of capnographs, mainstream and sidestream.

Mainstream is the arrangement where the analysing cell is interposed in the breathing system. This type do not cause turbulent flow in the breathing system nor do they extract gas from it (both of importance in paediatric anaesthesia) and they have a short delay time, but they are vulnerable to being dropped and damaged. They are also heavy and difficult to support when using a mask. They become hot and could burn patients.

Sidestream is where a continuous sample is drawn at the rate of (usually) 150 ml/min from the breathing system to be analysed within the machine. This is the more common arrangement, but the gas needs to be scavenged, or returned to the system if a circle is in use. Condensation forms and a water-trap is needed. It has a slower response time and is prone to diffusion errors and occlusion, however it is allows all the expensive parts of the system to be protected within a strong box which is important for prolonged reliability in the hurly-burly of the theatre environment.

Both require calibration before and at intervals during use against room air (presumed to have zero CO_2) and a occasional calibration against a standard gas mixture.

Proximal diversion is a compromise between mainstream and sidestream, where the analysing cell is distant from the monitor but not a part of the breathing system. It is supposed to combine the advantages, and diminish the disadvantages, of both arrangements.

••••••••••••••••••••••••••••••

10. HOW DO YOU MAKE SURE THAT A CAPNOGRAPH IS ACCURATE?

➡ **This is about calibration and zeroing**

Calibration is the verification of accuracy of measurement by comparison with a known concentration of the measured gas, usually 5.0% CO_2. The accuracy of most capnometers is 10% and the range is 0 - 10 kPa. Most capnometers do this automatically and one, the Nellcor Ultracap, is calibrated for life at the factory and needs no further calibration. *Zeroing* is that part of calibration where the reference is atmospheric, which actually consists of 0.03% CO_2. Drift is the tendency of the capnometer to deviate from the calibration values. This is most frequently due to accumulated secretions in the sampling tube.

The Belgian chemist van Helmont made and first described carbon dioxide in the 1620s but it was Joseph Black in 1754 who demonstrated that it was exhaled during breathing. It was briefly used as an anaesthetic in Wisconsin in 1928 by Henry Hill Hickman, without distinction; Luft identified infra-red absorption by CO_2 in 1943 and Elam and Liston developed clinical capnography in the 1950s.

••••••••••••••••••••••••••••••

11. WHAT IS CM$_5$ AND WHY IS IT BENEFICIAL?

➡ **This is a specific type of ECG lead placement. CM$_5$ is short for centri-manubrium-V$_5$, which describes the position of the two recording leads.**

In theatre use the ECG has three main uses:

1. Measurement of rate.
2. The detection and characterisation of arrhythmias.
3. The detection of myocardial ischaemia, characterised by ST-T wave changes.

The problem is that the best leads for visualising these various potential problems are as follows:

1. Arrhythmias are best seen in standard lead II that is orientated in the direction of the P-wave vector.
2. The detection of ischaemia depends on the vessel involved:
   - Left anterior descending artery (LAD) – V_1-V_4
   - Circumflex artery – V_4-V_6
   - Right coronary artery (inferior territory) – II, III, aVf.

In practice the best compromise in theatre is to combine II and V_5 as this allows monitoring of the rhythm and of ischaemia in the most important LAD territory. However in many monitoring systems it is impossible to easily monitor two leads so a modification of the two is used, the most popular being that described by Foex & Prys-Roberts in 1974 – CM$_5$.

••••••••••••••••••••••••••••••

12. WHAT PATTERNS MAY BE SEEN ON THE CAPNOGRAM AND WHAT DO THEY REPRESENT?

➡ **A diagram is useful. Begin by drawing the normal waveform.**

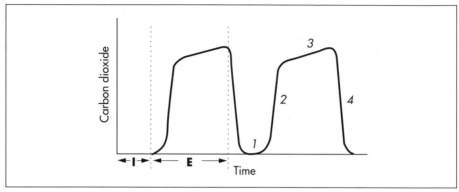

I = inspiration, E = expiration. The phases of the normal waveform are as follows.

1: Inspiration: should be at zero, since any elevation of the baseline indicates rebreathing. This is seen with the Mapleson D arrangement.

2: Upslope phase. If this is shallow, this indicates obstruction.

3: Plateau. This represents mixing of alveolar gas, and if sloped rather than flat, indicates uneven mixing, as in chronic airways disease.

4: Fall to zero at start of expiration.

These are some abnormal patterns:

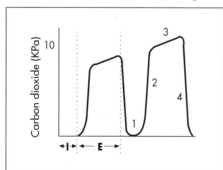

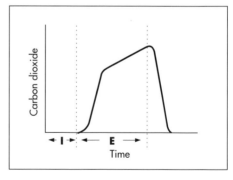

Malignant hyperpyrexia: High plateau PCO_2, rapid rate.

Chronic airways disease: Slow upstroke, wide $P(a\text{-}ET)CO_2$ gradient.

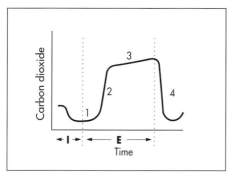

Defective valves in a circle system: Raised baseline with oscillations.

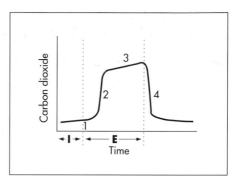

CO_2 rebreathing: Raised baseline.

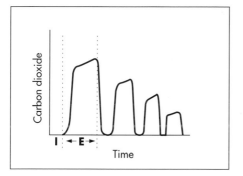

Reduced cardiac output: Progressive diminution in amplitude.

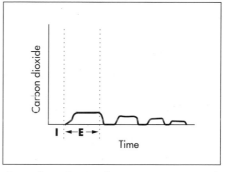

Oesophageal intubation: Even with carbonated drink in stomach, less than 6 deflections will be seen. Thereafter, the tube cannot be in the trachea if no CO_2 is detected, unless circulatory arrest has occurred.

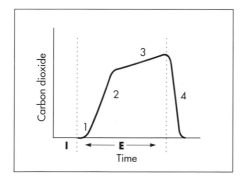

Airway obstruction: Slow ascent phase 2.

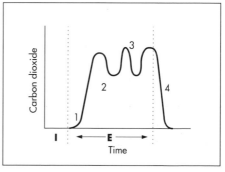

Recovery from neuromuscular blockade during positive pressure ventilation: Clefts are seen during phase 3.

13. WHAT IS THE ELECTRICAL EXPLANATION FOR ST ELEVATION ON THE ECG?

➡ **In order to explain this we have to explain exactly what we are seeing during the normal ECG tracing.**

The electrocardiogram measures the potential difference of the outside of the muscle membrane as the cardiac action potential passes along the fibres. Let us look at one schematic cardiac muscle fibre to explain the principle.

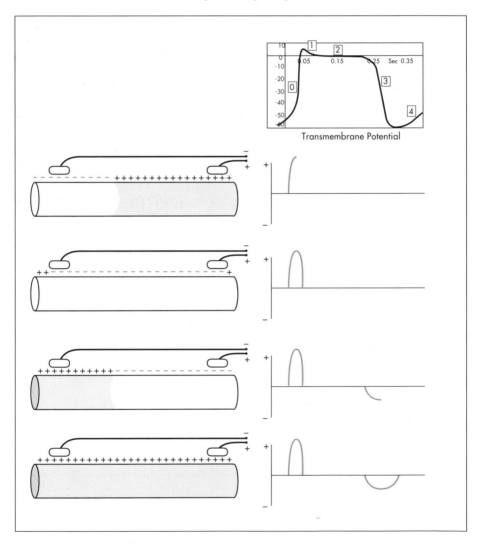

Transmembrane Potential

Initially as the depolarisation wave passes the first electrode there is a potential difference between the electrodes that is shown as a positive deflection of the recorder. This deflection then returns to zero as the depolarisation wave spreads to the second electrode. At this point there is no potential DIFFERENCE between the two electrodes (they are now both at the same negative potential, whereas before the wave started they were both at the same positive potential). As the recorder shows only potential difference there is no apparent difference between the two parts of the wave (PR and ST segments of the normal ECG). Finally the membrane repolarises a further deflection of the recorder. This is negative as the second electrode is initially negative relative to the first one. After repolarisation there is again no potential difference between the electrodes and so the record returns to zero. (Note that there is a range of time intervals before repolarisation is initiated in different ventricular fibres that explains the broadness of the T wave in relation to the QRS wave.)

Now let us consider what happens when there is a damaged segment of ventricular muscle that is unable to maintain polarisation (remembering that this is an energy-dependant active process). Thus at rest this part does not have a positive charge on its outside and so is at a negative potential compared with the rest of the heart. There is therefore current flow at rest, and this causes a negative deflection of the ECG between each beat – this is known as the current of injury. Depolarisation waves are seen as above, and now with the whole of the ventricle depolarised there is no current flow so the recorder returns to zero. The repolarisation wave is as before and during diastole the current of injury recurs.

It can therefore be seen that if we were able to calibrate the ECG such that we knew when there was zero current flow what we would see was not 'ST elevation' but negative deflection in diastole.

Finally it should be reiterated that the ECG baseline is neither the resting potential of the cardiac muscle or 0 mV, it is an indication of current flow.

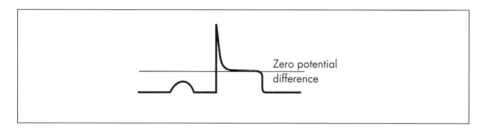

· ·

14. WHAT DISTORTIONS OCCUR WHEN USING PEN RECORDERS?

➡ **Pen recorders are valuable for displaying signals from patients that have a relatively low maximum frequency and produce a continuous and permanent paper record.**

The recorder consists of a heated needle or pen that is connected to a coil pivoted in the centre of a magnetic field. Changing the current through the coil alters its deflection which is resisted by a hair spring. This is the principle behind all galvanometers.

The distortions relate to two problems:

The inertia of the needle and its heating mechanism or ink means that it cannot respond to signals at a frequency of greater than about 80 Hz. Thus square wave changes lead to a sloping change in the record. In practice this is an adequate speed of response for ECG recording.

The needle is pivoted about a point so any square wave change will lead to an arced change on the record. Thus the maximum deflection is reduced (called sine distortion) and the timing of that maximum deflection will be distorted (timing error). These may be reduced by using paper that has a curved grid with a curvilinear deflection calibration.

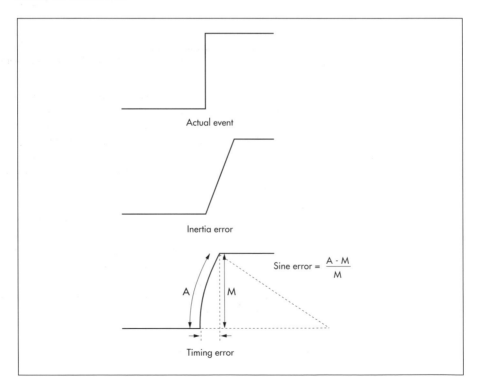

Actual event

Inertia error

$$\text{Sine error} = \frac{A - M}{M}$$

A M

Timing error

15. HOW IS TEMPERATURE MEASURED?

➡ **Temperature is a measure of the tendency of an object to gain or lose heat in contact with another object of different temperature. It is not a measure of the heat content or molecular excitation of an object.**

The techniques for measuring temperature are based on this definition of temperature, as heat will travel from a warmer object to a colder one until the temperature difference is eliminated.

The oldest form of thermometer as well as the most widely used is the mercury-in-glass thermometer. This relies on the principle that the mercury receives heat from the object and that its volume changes in proportion to that temperature change. It is effective in the range -39°C to ~250°C. If a thermometer is required for lower temperatures the alcohol-in-glass thermometer can be used (utilising the same principles) in the range -117°C to 78°C.

A wider range can be obtained by using gas thermometers which use the principles of the gas laws. The volume of a gas at fixed pressure (or the pressure of gas at fixed volume) alter proportionally to the change in temperature. Although inconvenient to use they have an effective range of -269°C to ~1600°C. They are generally used for calibration of other thermometers.

The Platinum Resistance Thermometer measures the change in electrical resistance of a length of pure platinum wire with change in temperature. The resistance increases with increasing temperature, but the change is not linear so calibration is required against a gas thermometer. It has a wide range (-250°C to ~1300°C).The resistance is then measured using a Wheatstone bridge (*see – **What is a Wheatstone bridge?***).

The thermistor is convenient for use in theatres. It is a semi-conductor device that has a reducing resistance with increasing temperature. Although the change is non-linear it can be manufactured so that over the working range (body temperature plus or minus 25°C) it is almost linear. Thermistors can also be made small enough that they are both fast responding and are convenient for clinical use. They do however tend to alter their characteristics over time ('drift') or if subjected to high temperatures (e.g. in an autoclave) so need recalibrating from time to time.

Another device seen in the laboratory is the thermocouple. This depends on the 'Seebeck effect'. When two conductors of different metals are connected together a potential difference is generated that is directly related to the temperature at the junction. If the circuit is the competed by another junction (the reference junction) the current produced is non-linearly related to the temperature difference between the two junctions. Thus if the temperature of the reference junction is known the temperature of the measurement junction can be measured. The measuring junction can be made very small and so have a very fast response and may be made in the form of a needle.

....

16. HOW DOES A CLARK ELECTRODE WORK?

➡️ **The Clark electrode is a polarographic electrode for measurement of the oxygen tension within a gas or liquid.**

The equipment consists of two electrodes - a platinum cathode and a silver/silver chloride anode. These are linked by a electrolyte medium containing potassium chloride. If a voltage (0.6V) is applied across the two electrodes the current that flows is proportional to the concentration of oxygen present, and thus this can be measured.

At the cathode each oxygen atom combines with four electrons to form four hydroxyl ions:

$$O_2 + 4e^- + 2H_2O \rightarrow 4OH^-$$

As the oxygen supply is rate-limiting the rate of reaction is proportional to it, and this is dependant on oxygen tension at the cathode. Hence the current flow is proportional to the oxygen tension.

The potassium chloride electrolytic medium is separated from the sample by a plastic membrane, and the oxygen tension equilibrates across the membrane. The electrode needs to be maintained at body temperature in order that the results are relevant.

The membrane may become coated with protein deposits or damaged and this can lead to inaccuracies.

••••••••••••••••••••••••••••••••

17. WHAT IS AN ISOBESTIC POINT?

➡️ **In any mixture of two gases a point at which the absorption coefficients are identical is called an isobestic point. The most important one in anaesthetic practice is at 800nm seen in a mixture of the oxygenated and deoxygenated forms of haemoglobin.**

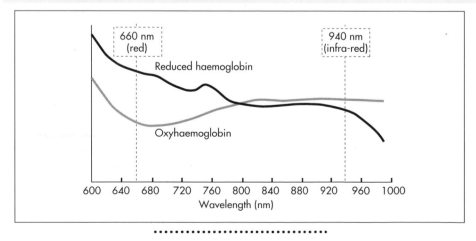

••••••••••••••••••••••••••••••••

18. HOW DOES THE OSCILLOTONOMETER WORK

➡ **The oscillotonometer uses two cuffs, one to occlude arteria and one to sense pulsations and amplify them by a sensitive aneroid chamber.**

The oscillotonometer (eponymously known as Von Recklinghausen's oscillotonometer) consists of a double cuff, an inflating bulb, two separate aneroid capsules within a sealed unit, a lever and a dial. The upper (proximal) cuff is the occluding cuff and is 5 cm wide, the lower (distal) is the sensing cuff and is 10 cm wide. The two cuffs overlap. The coarse aneroid chamber is sealed and responds to changes in pressure within the sealed case, which it transmits to a gauge by means of a rack and pinion device. The sensitive chamber is connected to the distal, sensing cuff. The lever operates in two positions. In position 1, which is the default position, the inflating bulb communicates with both cuffs. In position 2, there is a communication between the sensitive capsule and the sensing cuff, and the pressure relief valve allows the cuffs to deflate.

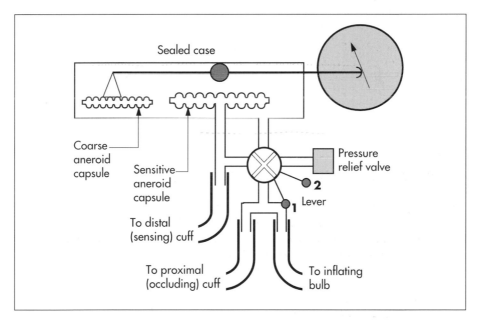

The system is inflated with the manual bulb. Both cuffs inflate to the same pressure, which is in continuity with the inside of the sealed case. The coarse chamber is compressed and the pressure indicated on the gauge, since the two are connected by a rack and pinion device. Once inflated above systolic, the lever is moved to position 2. As the occluding cuff deflates, pulsations will reach the sensing cuff and fluctuations will occur in the sensitive capsule. The fluctuations distort the sensitive chamber, changing the pressure within the sealed case. These pulsations are transmitted to the gauge. Oscillations will appear at systolic pressure, become maximal at mean arterial pressure, and disappear at diastolic pressure.

. . . .

19. HOW DOES A PULSE OXIMETER WORK AND WHAT ARE THE PROBLEMS ASSOCIATED WITH ITS USE?

➡️ **The pulse oximeter relies on measurement of the different absorption of oxyhaemoglobin and deoxyhaemoglobin at two different wavelengths.**

The oximeter emits pulses of infrared (940 nm) and red (660 nm) light every 5 to 10 μsec. It then aims to identify the points of maximum (systole) and minimum (diastole) absorption. It measures the pulsatile component of the absorption at each of the two wavelengths and subtracts the constant component (i.e. that part that is not due to arterial blood). It then compares the absorption at the two different wavelengths and compares the ratio to an algorithm calculated from experimental data. The oxygenated haemoglobin absorbs more infrared light and less red light than the deoxygenated molecule. (See graph: *What is an isobestic point?*)

Pulse oximetry is most accurate above 90% oxyhaemoglobin saturation, and much less accurate below 70%. The machines are calibrated against healthy volunteers, which makes calibration to values below 70% ethically unacceptable.

Error in calculating the pulsatile component of the light absorption

- Failure due to low pulse pressure, vasoconstriction, hypotension and venous pulsation.

    All these make it harder for the oximeter to define the points of maximum and minimum absorption (systole and diastole).

- Interference from abnormal haemoglobins (e.g. carboxyhaemoglobin or methaemoglobin) or intravenous dyes (e.g. methylene blue, indocyanine green)

    These will all affect the pulsatile component and so are entered in the machine's calculation of the saturation. The functional saturation (ratio of oxygenated haemoglobin to haemoglobin that is available for oxygenation) is therefore altered. Bilirubin absorption is similar to that of deoxygenated haemoglobin and so gives a falsely-low reading for HbO. Carboxyhaemoglobin, which has an absorption is similar to oxyhaemoglobin, will give a misleadingly high reading for HbO. Methaemoglobin, which has an absorption that is similar at the two wavelengths monitored tends to produce a SpO_2 that approaches 85%. Fetal haemoglobin has no effect.

- Irregular pulse rate

    Atrial fibrillation and other arrhythmias make it harder for the machine to predict the points of maximum and minimum absorption.

Increase of the ratio of the non-pulsatile component of the light absorption.

- Nail varnish and dirt or staining on fingers

    These tend to increase the non-pulsatile absorption and so will make the pulsatile component relatively small and less sensitive.

- Optical interference

  Light from room lights especially if it is flickering (and so 'pulsatile') can affect the SpO_2. Normally in excess ambient light the oximeter will fail to provide a reading, and the probe should be shielded.

Machine dysfunction

- Electrical interference

  Diathermy will affect the reading circuitry in the oximeter and this normally causes loss of the reading, and occasionally inaccurate pulse rates.

Other problems relate to the physiology of oxygen saturation

- Saturation is of little value in assessing high oxygen tensions

  Because of the shape of the haemoglobin dissociation curve the oximeter is unable to differentiate high but safe oxygen tensions from those that may be excessive and risk toxicity.

- Oximetry is a poor monitor of ventilatory or airway failure

  Arterial oxygenation is a late indicator of hypoventilation or failure of the airway (e.g. oesophageal intubation) and must not be relied on as a monitor of this.

Finally it should be noted that oximeters may be a danger to the patient:

- There are a number of reports of pressure damage especially in those patients monitored for prolonged periods with low peripheral perfusion pressures.
- A number of patients have suffered burns from the probe, either due to incompatibility in probe and monitor or when some oximeters are used in MRI scanners.

······························

20. HOW DO YOU MEASURE BLOOD PRESSURE?

➡ **Blood pressure can be measured invasively, which involves cannulating an artery, or non-invasively.**

Invasive blood pressure monitoring

This may be performed at any accessible peripheral artery, the radial being the most popular. The risk to the vessel patency increases with the duration of cannulation. A 20G teflon cannula is used. The other requirements are:

1. A column of fluid in a short (less than 120 cm), wide-bore (1.5–3.0 mm internal diameter), rigid tube free from air. If the tubing is too long, resonance will occur; if compliant, or if air is in the system, there will be excessive damping of the signal.
2. A pressure transducer. This converts energy in one form (pressure), into another (electricity).
3. Amplifier and signal-processor.
4. Display. This may be on a cathode ray tube, or on a digital readout, or commonly both. The advantage of the latter arrangement is that accurate numerical data is combined with a visual impression of the waveform, allowing other information to be derived from it.

The advantages of invasive monitoring are:

1. Continuous information, on a beat-to-beat basis. Non-invasive blood pressure (NIBP) measurement can be repeated only up to once a minute, as this is the interval the machine requires to take the measurement.
2. Continuous measurement is more accurate.
3. Other information can be derived from the signal:
   - Heart rate
   - Stroke volume, from the area under the curve.
   - Contractility, from the gradient of the up-slope.
   - Resistance and compliance of the arterial tree, from the diastolic delay.
   - Myocardial work and O_2 consumption, which is proportional to the area under the curve of systolic pressure and time.
   - Myocardial perfusion, which is proportional to the area under the curve of diastolic pressure and time.
   - The effect of any dysrhythmia is immediately apparent from the amplitude of the pressure wave corresponding to the abnormal QRS complex.
     Invasive monitoring of blood pressure was first performed by a clergyman, Stephen Hales, on a conscious horse using a column of water in 1733.

Non-invasive blood pressure monitoring

This may be performed as follows:

1. Use of a Riva-Rocci cuff and auscultation of the Korotkoff sounds (*See* – **What is the principle behind the Riva-Rocci cuff and Korotkoff sounds and why may they be inaccurate?**)

2. Use of an automated blood pressure machine (*See* – **What is the most accurate measurement on the dinamap?**)

3. By an oscillotonometer. (*See* – **How does the oscillotonometer work?**)

....

21. WHAT IS PARAMAGNETISM?

➡ **Paramagnetism is said of a gas which is attracted to a magnetic field and is the opposite of diamagnetic, which is to be repelled by a magnetic field. It is a principle employed in oxygen analysis.**

Oxygen (and nitric oxide) are paramagnetic whereas other gases tend to be diamagnetic. This is due to the configuration of the electrons in the outer shell of the molecules. A differential pressure transducer is suspended between the sample gas, containing oxygen of

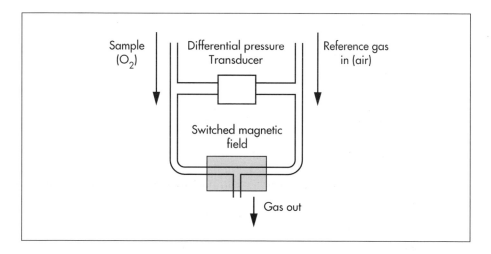

unknown concentration, and a reference gas, which is air, and has a known oxygen concentration. A strong pulsed magnetic field is applied over the junction of the two gases. There will then be a correspondingly pulsed pressure change between the two tubes if there is a difference in the oxygen concentration, and hence the paramagnetic tendency, of the two samples. The pressure difference can then be calibrated against different oxygen concentrations.

This is used in the Datex oxygen analyser. The response is rapid, but the equipment is expensive.

....

22. WHAT IS THE PIEZO-ELECTRIC EFFECT?

➡ **The piezo-electric effect is the property of a substance which, when it is exposed to pressure, generates an electric charge.**

This effect implies the presence of a transducer, and is the basis of ultrasound. Ultrasound is generated by employing the piezo-electric effect in reverse, in other words a high frequency voltage is applied to a crystal which then oscillates at the frequency of the applied potential difference; this generates ultrasound radiation. The ultrasound transducer performs two tasks; it generates and transmits ultrasound radiation, and it also senses the returned signal. The returned ultrasound signal is again transduced into electrical energy and displayed as an image.

➡ **This leads on to the next question:**

•••••••••••••••••••••••••••••••

23. HOW DOES ULTRASOUND WORK?

➡ **Ultrasound detects soft tissue interfaces by the reflection of ultrasound radiation.**

Waves in water oscillate at right angles to the direction of travel of the wave. Sound waves by contrast are transmitted by oscillation of particles in the direction of propagation of the wave;

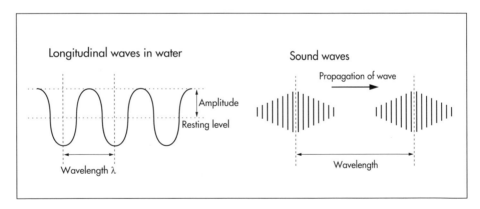

The speed at which the wave moves is $c = \lambda f$ where the wavelength is denoted by λ, and the frequency by f, which determines the pitch of the sound; the amplitude of the wave determines the loudness. Ultrasound is sound whose pitch (i.e., frequency) is above that audible to the human ear; this is above 20,000 Hz, although clinical ultrasound operates between 1 and 10 MHz, some 50,000 times higher than the audible range; I wondered if dogs might hear ultrasound, but in light of this I think not, although bats and dolphins operate at up to 100 KHz.

Ultrasound is absorbed by tissues (attenuation) and reflected by tissue interfaces. The extent to which the signal is attenuated depends on the nature of the tissue and on the frequency of the radiation. Bone and air have the highest attenuation coefficients, and water the smallest; this is why ultrasound travels badly through air-filled cavities such as gut and lung, and why a full bladder is used as a window for ultrasound imaging of the gravid uterus. There is a balance to be struck between penetration of tissues and resolution of images. The lowest frequency ultrasound achieves the highest tissue penetration, but low frequency implies long wavelength as the two are inversely related:

$$f = \frac{c}{\lambda}$$

Long wavelength is associated with lower resolution. The solution is to use ultrasound of the highest frequency (and shortest wavelength, and best resolution) that will just penetrate tissue adequately. This in turn depends on the nature of the tissue, so 3-5 MHz is used for abdominal scanning and 10 MHz for the eye.

Wavelength of ultrasound used in the human:

Sound travels through tissue at 1500 m/sec. For 10 MHz ultrasound, taking $c = \lambda f$, $1500 = \lambda \times 10,000,000$

The wavelength of ultrasound used in the human must be $1500/10,000,000 = 0.0015$ m $= 0.15$ mm.

•••••••••••••••••••••••••••••••

24. WHAT MODES OF ULTRASOUND HAVE YOU SEEN IN USE?

➡ **There are A-scans, B-scans, M-mode scans, and realtime. Of these, A and B are largely historical and it is M-mode and realtime which are the terms of interest. You might then mention Doppler ultrasound, or you might be asked about it, although it does not fit into the classification above.**

A-scan:

From *amplitude* scan. This is the simplest type, and reflection of ultrasound radiation is used to determine depth, as a delay in return of the signal of 1 microsecond corresponds to a distance to tissue interface of 0.75 mm.

B-scan:

From *brightness* modulation. The intensity of the returned signal is displayed in a proportionally bright image.

M-Mode:

From *movement* mode. This is a B-scan with a display produced against time. This allows for the creation of a two-dimensional image, and is used in echocardiography.

Realtime:

An instrument which produces and displays an image at more than 20 frames a second is said to be operating in realtime. Realtime scanners use pulsed ultrasound, where the radiation is transmitted, a latent period ensues to allow the reverberations to die down, and there is then a further period when the reverberations return to the transducer. This takes 300 microseconds. The rate of repetition of this process, and therefore of generation of the image, is constrained by the speed at which the ultrasound travels. One pulse contributes one line of a B-scan; 100 lines are needed to generate an image. The maximal pulse repetition is 3000/second, which means that 30 images can be created per second. This exceeds the 20 frames a second necessary to create a realtime picture.

Realtime scanning is used for obstetric ultrasound and other diagnostic abdominal and thoracic ultrasound. Invasive (transoesophageal and transcervical) ultrasound also depends on realtime technology.

••••••••••••••••••••••••••••••••

25. WHAT IS DOPPLER ULTRASOUND?

➡ **In 1842 Christian Doppler (an Austrian physicist) discovered that the shift in the reflected frequency of an optic wave is proportional to the velocity at which the reflecting object is moving.**

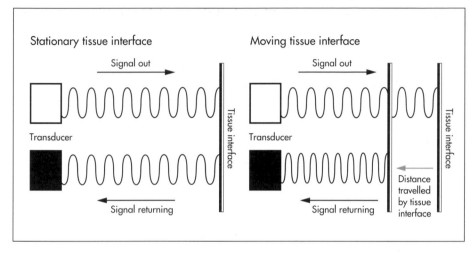

The principle can be thought of by first imagining the wave reflected off a still mirror and then measuring the frequency of the peaks of the waves as they hit the mirror, and so as they reach the receiver. Now if the mirror is moving towards the waves then the wave peaks will reach the mirror quicker and be reflected as a wave with the peaks closer together and so a higher frequency. This change can be displayed audibly or visually, using colour to indicate velocity. The wave used is of ultrasonic frequency, and the frequency is adjusted to change the depth at which measurements are made (high frequencies are for superficial measurements whereas lower frequencies allow deeper measurement).

Doppler ultrasound is used in adult echocardiography, in fetal echocardiography, and in the measurement of uterine artery flow. In vascular surgery it is used to confirm the of patency of vessels. It may also be used to measure blood pressure by detection of vessel wall motion.

A Duplex scanner is one which combines realtime ultrasound with Doppler imaging.

The velocity of the blood is calculated by referring to the equation:

$$\text{Velocity} = \frac{\delta f \cdot V_{sound}}{2f \cdot \cos \theta}$$

where:

δf = Doppler shift in frequency

V_{sound} = Velocity of sound in tissue

f = Initial frequency of the ultrasound wave

θ = Incident angle of the beam to the blood movement. If this is less than 30% then $\cos \theta$ approximates to 1.

• •

26. HOW DOES MAGNETIC RESONANCE IMAGING WORK?

➡ **Magnetic resonance imaging (MRI) depends on absorption of electro-magnetic radiation by, and emission of radiofrequency radiation from, atomic nuclei.**

MRI was originally known as nuclear magnetic resonance, which I think is a better term; however the word "nuclear" was removed to alleviate concerns about ionising radiation, which does not feature in the technique.

Every proton in an atomic nucleus has a single positive charge. Protons act in pairs, so that each having opposite spin characteristics, they cancel out. In an atom with an odd number of protons, (H^+, ^{13}C) one proton will be unpaired and will have spin and charge. Normally this is irrelevant, but if exposed to an electromagnetic field the nucleus containing an unpaired proton will align itself along the axis of the magnetic field. When the electromagnetic field is withdrawn, the atomic nucleus reverts to its original position, and in so doing, releases energy as radio waves. The energy involved is very small, so MRI can only be used to detect substances present in at least millimolar concentrations.

MRI can be used to define anatomy in axial computed tomography, like the Xray-based equivalent, but with better views of the soft tissues and in particular the posterior fossa of the skull. MRI can also perform spectroscopic analysis of biochemical processes.

T_1 and T_2 refer to the relaxation time constants, where T_2 is the spin–spin relaxation constant, the time taken for the decay of the signal. T_1 is the spin–lattice relaxation time.

Magnetic field strengths:

The magnetic field strengths used in MRI are considerable. The earth's magnetic field is of the order of 1 Gauss; 1 tesla (1T) = 10,000 Gauss. The fields in MRI scanners are between 0.05 and 2.0 tesla. Around the machine there will be a measurable fringe field, within which ferromagnetic items (bleeps, needles, stethoscopes, gas cylinders) may be subjected to movement but which will also distort the image generated by the machine. The fringe field may be defined in terms of the 50 Gauss and 5 Gauss lines; these lie about 8 m from the machine, or less depending on the shielding on the equipment.

•••••••••••••••••••••••••••••••

27. WHAT ARE THE PROBLEMS PERFORMING ANAESTHESIA FOR MRI SCANNING?

➡ **This is about the enclosed space of an MRI scanner (smaller space than a conventional CT) and the intrusion into the powerful electromagnetic field.**

- Sedation is often required because the MRI environment is extremely claustrophobic. Children and anxious adults may need to be anaesthetised for scanning to take place, which may take up to an hour - this is longer than for a conventional CT.
- Access to the anaesthetised patient is a concern because of the enclosed space and because of the delay in extracting the patient from the machine should it become necessary.
- Regarding the effects of the magnetic field:
  - Ferromagnetic objects will be subjected to force sufficient to move them in fields over 50 Gauss, and so must be placed outside the marked 50 Gauss line.
  - Infusion devices fail in fields over 100 Gauss.
  - Pacemakers fail in fields over 5 Gauss.
  - Electric cable may have a current induced within it by the magnet and heat up as a consequence. Cabling must be minimised and where present, insulated.

•••••••••••••••••••••••••••••••

28. HOW DO YOU CONDUCT ANAESTHESIA SAFELY FOR MRI?

➡ **In anaesthesia for CT, the anaesthetic machine and the monitoring can be there, but the anaesthetist cannot; in anaesthesia for MRI, the anaesthetist can be there but the equipment cannot.**

- *Induction:* Conventional, performed outside the magnetic field.
- *Airway:* RAE polar tracheal tube, which contours snugly around the face and connects to a breathing system, which should be a coaxial arrangement at least 10 m long.
- *Maintenance*: Spontaneous respiration or manual IPPV with the anaesthetic machine outside the 50 Gauss line. There are nonmagnetic anaesthetic machines available, which include aluminium cylinders. Volatiles and total intravenous techniques have both been used.
- *Monitoring*: The dorsalis pedis pulse may be accessible. An oesophageal stethoscope is useful. Capnography with extended tubing is possible, but the delay time is extended. ECG electrodes cannot be used.
- *Reversal*: Remove the patient from the field before allowing them to wake up.

•••••••••••••••••••••••••••••••

29. HOW CAN DEPTH OF ANAESTHESIA BE MEASURED?

➡ **One of the principle requirements of general anaesthesia is that the patient should not have any recall of events whilst they are anaesthetised. The risk of recall should be inversely related to the depth of anaesthesia.**

Depth of anaesthesia is notoriously difficult to measure accurately.

Measurements of depth rely on:

Clinical Monitoring
(normally autonomic effects; but may be affected by drugs or disease)

- **Pupil size**

  Decrease with increasing depth, but pupils may dilate at very deep levels.

- **Cardiovascular changes**

  BP and HR decrease with increased depth, though this depends on the agent used (e.g. ketamine or cyclopropane tend to maintain BP) and may be altered by other drugs that do not affect depth of anaesthesia. Furthermore alterations in physiology (e.g. haemorrhage or hypercarbia) have profound effects on cardiovascular parameters.

- **Sweating and lacrimation**

  Both MAY indicate light anaesthesia, but may be present at adequate depth. Lacrimation seems to be more reliable as a measure of depth.

- **Combinations of these**

  Various clinical scoring systems have been developed to try to quantify these parameters (e.g. the PRST system) but the problems inherent in the individual measures are still present if they are grouped together.

Response to command

- **The isolated forearm technique**

  A tourniquet is placed on the arm before neuromuscular blockage commences, so it is possible to keep part of the patient unparalysed. However it is only of value for 20 minutes as ischaemic paralysis sets in at this stage, and investigation into recall and depth of anaesthesia using this technique has been inconclusive.

- **Instrumental Monitoring**

  (these are divided into machines that measure autonomic and other functions that may be related to depth of anaesthesia or to neurological background activity, and those that direct measure cerebral electrical activity)

- **Skin conductance**

  This is a quantified measure of sweating.

- **Digital plethysmography**

  Measures sympathetic activity by measuring the amplitude of the pulsatile fluctuations in finger volume that occur with systolic blood flow. If the amplitude falls this suggests vasoconstriction that may be due to lightening anaesthesia.

- **Lower oesophageal contractility**

  The lower oesophageal sphincter is smooth muscle and therefore free of the effects of neuromuscular blocking agents. It has been found that there is a non-propulsive rhythmic contraction that occurs in this area (duration 2-5 seconds, frequency 5 or more per minute). This is known as tertiary activity and is suppressed by anaesthetic agents in an apparently dose-related manner. However the activity is altered by many other factors including disease states, type of surgery and other drugs, as well as having a with inter-individual variability.

- **Ocular microtremor**

- **EMG**

- **R-R beat-to-beat variability**

  There has been some effort in equating the variability of the R-R interval with depth of anaesthesia, but this has rather fallen out of favour now.

- **Electroencephalogram**

  In order to use the EEG it must first be processed in an attempt to filter out unnecessary information and leave behind a simple score that may be related to depth of anaesthesia. Not only is this difficult it also may be logically flawed as the EEG demonstrated the activity of the cerebral cortex whereas most anaesthetic agents are believed to act deeper within the brain. The methods that have been used for processing include:

  a) *Cerebral function monitor* (CFM) - this displays total amplitude in the 2-20Hz range but maybe better for assessing cerebral oxygenation than depth of anaesthesia.

  b) *Compressed spectral array* - this displays the amplitude at varying frequencies (Fourier analysis), however this is still too complex to be of use.

  c) *Spectral edge* - this measures the frequency below which 95% of the total EEG power occurs (or the 95th centile).

  d) *Cerebral function analysing monitor* (CFAM) - a development of the CFM that displays the information in the different frequency bands of the EEG waves (alpha to delta).

  As can be seen from the multiple EEG methods there is presently no obvious candidate that is easy to use, repeatable and accurate.

- **Evoked potentials**

  Auditory, visual and somatosensory potentials have been used. The advantage of there methods is that it may measure activity deep within the brain, and furthermore there is evidence that the changes induced by deepening anaesthesia can be reversed by surgical stimuli, suggesting that this is not merely an assay of cerebral anaesthetic concentration.

  Presently the most promising method would appear to be early cortical auditory evoked potentials, although this is expensive, prone to interference from other equipment and not devoid of changes with altering physiology (especially temperature and pCO_2).

....

30. HOW DO YOU MONITOR THE NEUROMUSCULAR JUNCTION?

➡ **You should describe the nerve stimulator: this delivers 50 mA for 0.2 - 1.0 msec, and requires 50 - 300 V. It is applied over the course of a mixed peripheral nerve, which it then stimulates while the anaesthetist observes muscle function in the distribution of the nerve. The nerve stimulator is therefore a monitor of the neuromuscular junction.**

Fout tests are used to detect type of, degree of, reversibility of, and recovery from, neuromuscular block.

Twitch-tetanus-twitch

This distinguishes the *type* of block; four patterns are observed.

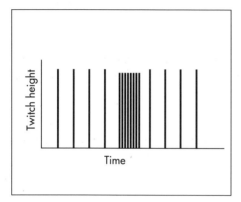

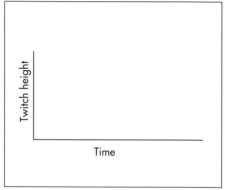

Normal; symmetrical twitches followed by sustained tetanic contraction; no post-tetanic facilitation (PTF).

Total block; no response.

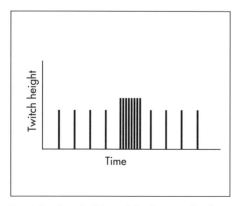

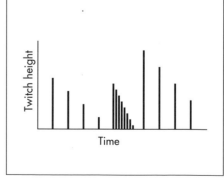

Partial depolarising block; weak but symmetrical twitches, sustained tetanic contraction, no PTF.

Partial non-depolarising block; weak twitches, fade on tetanic stimulus, post-tetanic facilitation.

Train of four

This distinguishes the *degree* of block. It is possible to use the count, or the ratio of force of 4th to 1st twitch ($T_4:T_1$).

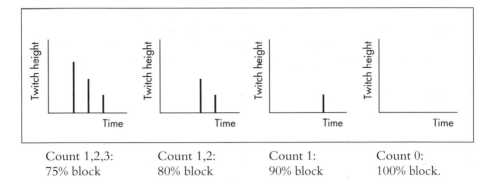

Count 1,2,3: Count 1,2: Count 1: Count 0:
75% block 80% block 90% block 100% block.

Post-tetanic twitch count

This determines the *reversibility* of a non-depolarising block; the device delivers 50 Hz for 5 sec, then 1 Hz, counting detectable twitches. Reversal is possible if count is greater than 10.

Double burst

This uses a pair of bursts of 3 pulses at 50 Hz pulses separated by 0.75 sec. It assesses *recovery* from non-depolarising block, displaying the $T_1:T_4$ ratio.

· ·

31. WHAT ARE THE CHARACTERISTIC COMPONENTS OF THE CVP TRACE AND WHAT AFFECTS THEM?

➡️ **There are three waves (a, c and v) and two descents (x and y)**

a wave

- This is produced by the contraction of the right atrium (atrial systole). It is therefore absent in atrial fibrillation. It is increased by anything that impedes right atrial emptying (tricuspid or pulmonary stenosis, right ventricular hypertrophy, pulmonary hypertension). Heart block leads to variable A waves, and complete heart block may lead to 'cannon' waves when the right atrial contracts against the closed tricuspid valve.

c wave

- This occurs just after the onset of ventricular systole and is caused by the leaflets of the tricuspid valve bulging into the right atrium during the initial isovolumetric ventricular contraction.

v wave

- This is caused by the filling of the right atrium against the closed tricuspid valve. In tricuspid incompetence it is increased by the back flow of blood from the right ventricle during ventricular systole and so will be very prominent.

x descent

- This is the result of the relaxation of the atrium and the downward movement of the tricuspid leaflets as the ventricle contracts during the ejection phase. It does not occur if the tricuspid valve is incompetent.

y descent

- This occurs when the tricuspid valve opens and blood flows from the right atrium to the right ventricle.
- After the **y descent** there is a small deflection in the ascending limb of the **a wave**, this is due to the completion of passive ventricular filling, is known as the **h wave**. This can normally only be seen in bradycardia.

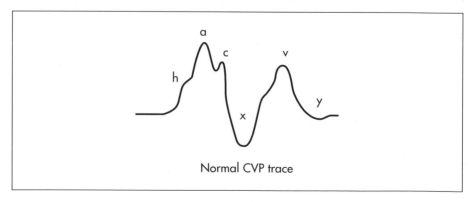

Normal CVP trace

32. HOW DO YOU MEASURE FUNCTIONAL RESIDUAL CAPACITY?

➡ **Functional residual capacity (FRC) is the lung volume in which gas exchange takes place.**

A drawing or the spirometry is very useful, and demonstrates that you at least know what FRC represents.

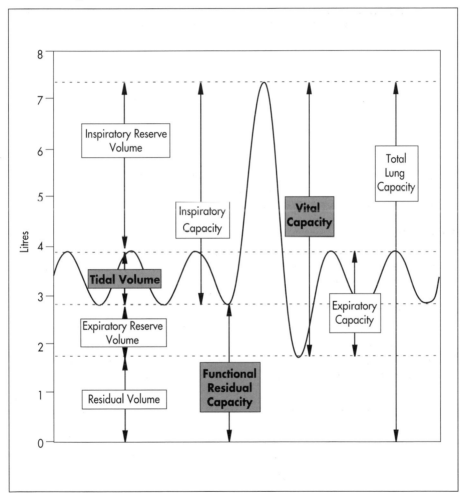

There are at least two methods to measure FRC.

Helium dilution:

This involves breathing an oxygen-enriched gas mixture with a known concentration of helium, from a circle system with a carbon dioxide absorber. Helium is not taken up by the circulation, and so if the volume of the apparatus is known, and the final concentration of helium is measured, this allows measurement of total lung capacity.

$[He]_{Initial} \times Vol_{equip} = [He]_{equilibrium} \times Vol_{(equipment + total lung capacity)}.$

One can derive residual volume and FRC, by using spirometry and arithmetic. However Helium dilution cannot measure that volume which is behind closed airways, because the helium cannot get there.

Body plethysmograph:

In order to measure FRC in, for example, a patient with emphysema and airway closure, the body plethysmograph must be used. This uses Boyle's law, $P1 \times V1 = P2 \times V2$.

....

33. WHAT IS THE PRINCIPLE BEHIND THE 'RIVA-ROCCI' CUFF AND KOROTKOFF SOUNDS AND HOW MAY THEY BE INACCURATE?

➡ **The Riva–Rocci (named after an Italian doctor) cuff was first described as a measurement of blood pressure one hundred years ago in 1896. Initially the systolic pressure was determined by palpation; Nikolai Korotkoff reported an auscultatory method in 1905.**

The Riva–Rocci cuff is the eponymous name for the blood pressure cuff and the Korotkoff sounds are the noises heard over the brachial artery during deflation of an occluding proximal cuff and are taken as measurements of blood pressure.

Korotkoff originally described three sounds; five are now described.

- Phase I: Appearance of a tapping sound, corresponding to the systolic pressure.
- Phase II: Muffling or disappearance of sounds; "auscultatory gap".
- Phase III: Sounds reappear.
- Phase IV: Sounds become muffled again. This is taken as diastolic pressure in the UK.
- Phase V: Sounds disappear.

Although there is no definite answer to what causes the sounds it seems reasonable to assume that the sounds are created by turbulent flow causing vibration of the arterial wall, and the sound is subsequently amplified and transmitted through the tissues to the stethoscope. When the pressure within the vessel changes as the systolic pulsation passes it reaches a point when the pressure difference across the vessel wall is zero. This is highly conductive to vessel wall vibration and so the vibrations are heard when the cuff pressure is between systolic and diastolic pressures.

There is some discussion as to whether Korotkoff phase IV (sudden muffling of the sounds) or phase V (disappearance of the sounds) should be used for the diastolic pressure. Both slightly over-read in comparison with direct methods (phase IV more so), but phase V is said to be a gradual process and so the exact point is difficult to determine, and in high output states (such as pregnancy) phase V may not occur until the cuff is fully deflated.

Errors in the reading of blood pressure relate to:

Cuff width - A narrow cuff will give an overly high reading and a wide cuff too low a reading. The cuff width is said to need to be 2/3 of the length of the fore-arm.

Cuff length - The inflating part of the cuff must lie over the artery so that the pressure within the cuff is the same as the pressure that is transmitted to the vessel wall.

Aneroid gauges - Errors in the zeroing and calibration of these gauges are common causes of error in their use.

Atherosclerosis - The vessel walls tend to be stiffer and so the vibration is reduced, and its frequency may fall below the audible range, making the sounds dfficult to hear.

Hypotension - Sounds become much more difficult to hear.

• •

3 QUESTIONS ON CLINICAL ANAESTHESIA

HOW WOULD YOU ANAESTHETISE...?

Questions on clinical cases are under-represented in this book. This is deliberate. The answer to these questions at Primary level relate strongly to the individual experience of the junior anaesthetist. Candidates should remember that the examiners do not expect them to have seen or done every procedure and there is no shame in answering the question "Have you seen a ...?" with "No, but from my reading I understand that...". This is much better than saying yes then displaying that you either have not seen or were not concentrating during that case. It goes without saying that there are some cases that examiners will be surprised if you have not come across.

➡ **The structure of the answer is constant and should consist of:**

Preoperative visit

- *a.* History & examination (with reference to points specific to the case)
- *b.* Investigations required and results expected
- *c.* Premedication prescribed (not just analgesic or sedative)
- *d.* Resuscitation measures if required

Pre-Anaesthetic

- *a.* Assistance (both senior and ODA)
- *b.* IV access
- *c.* Monitoring
- *d.* Equipment (and checking)

Anaesthetic

- *a.* (The technique that the candidate is most familiar with is generally the best)
- *b.* Induction
- *c.* Airway and ventilation
- *d.* Maintenance
- *e.* Expected anaesthetic & surgical problems
- *f.* Reversal & recovery

Post-Operative

a. Orders for the nursing staff

b. Analgesia

c. Other Medication

d. Fluid Management

e. Oxygen

The important point to note is that the answer does not just consist of "I would give thiopentone, atracurium and fentanyl, followed by intubation and maintenance of anaesthesia with oxygen, nitrous oxide and isoflurane". Indeed in many cases the actual drugs used are just a matter of personal preference and it is the pre-operative management that is of interest.

Finally when selecting a technique for the particular anaesthetic candidates should consider their own experience. The examiner may feel that he would anaesthetise an ASA 4, 93 year old lady with a fractured neck of femur using a 3-in-1 block with local infiltration and a propofol infusion for sedation but if *you* are more experienced with a general anaesthetic then this (after saying that you would call for senior assistance) is the technique that is safest in *your* hands.

•••••••••••••••••••••••••••••••

1. WHAT IS THE DIFFERENCE BETWEEN A NEONATE AND A CHILD?

➡ **A neonate is defined as being less than 45 weeks post-conception, regardless of age from birth.**

➡ **This is a very general question and offers the opportunity to divert the viva into an area of good knowledge. Some pointers to this are given below.**

Respiratory considerations

A neonate has smaller air passages, will be an obligate nose-breather (and thus highly susceptible to obstruction) with a high glottis, at level of C4. A neonate will have a resting oxygen consumption at least twice that of an adult; 6.8 ml/kg/min. This means hypoxia will occur twice as quickly as in an adult. A 3 mm internal diameter, 12 cm length tracheal tube is the one with which to start. There will be no cuff on this tube; a leak is essential – it ensures that the mucosa will not be compressed and rendered ischaemic. If the leak is too great, or if airway contamination is a risk, a pharyngeal pack can be used. It is usual to hand-ventilate with a fresh gas flow of at least 3.0 L/min, using the Jackson-Rees modification of Ayre's t-piece.

Cardiovascular considerations

Cardiac output is rate-dependant as the myocardium is rich in mitochondria and incompliant. Normal heart rate is 120 - 140 bpm, and normal systolic pressure is 80 mmHg. These are both relatively well preserved in hypovolaemia, but sudden decompensation is a feature. Cardiac index is normally high (4.8 - 5.0 l/min/m^2). Venous engorgement of the liver is an important sign of fluid overload or right-sided failure.

Beware the transitional circulation. This is the re-establishment of the foetal circulation following an episode of hypoxia and reopening of the ductus arteriosus. It cannot occur after four weeks post delivery as the ductus has closed permanently by this stage.

Normal haemoglobin at birth is 17 -22 g/dl, consisting of both in the fetal form haemoglobin (HbF) and the adult form.

Metabolic considerations

Hypoglycaemia is the main risk as glycogen reserves are small and metabolic rate is high. Thus feeding should not be withheld for any time greater than 3 hours, unless substituted by intravenous route. There is rapid redistribution within a small volume of distribution – thus $t_{1/2}\alpha$ is short, but accumulation will occur. There is limited renal and hepatic clearance of drugs and metabolites.

....

2.   WHAT ARE THE INDICATIONS FOR TRACHEOSTOMY?

➡️ **These may be divided into four groups. Laryngectomy, surgical removal of the larynx, results in a tracheostome.**

To bypass obstruction above the level of the trachea

Wheeze causes an expiratory sound, whereas stridor is an inspiratory sound. An important cause of stridor is epiglottitis, which may occur in the adult.

To separate passage of food and air

This is important where the complicated neurological mechanism which normally allows for separate passage of food and air is impaired, for example in neurological injury or degenerative disease; aspiration would otherwise occur.

To allow repeated aspiration and clearance of secretions

This is necessary where normal clearance mechanisms have failed. Mini-tracheostomy has shortcomings, mostly in that a suction catheter cannot generate displacement of secretions where it fits tightly into a small tracheostomy - there needs to be a passage of air around it.

To allow prolonged controlled ventilation

The commonest indication on ITU. There is considerable debate surrounding the ideal time to perform a tracheostomy, opinion dividing between early and late.

•••••••••••••••••••••••••••••••

3. WHAT ARE THE FEATURES AND BENEFITS OF THE 'TEC 5 SERIES OF VAPORISERS?

➡ **You should know the design and advantages of the vaporiser that you use.**

The 'Tec series are the most common vaporisers in the UK and the 'Tec 5 series is at the time of writing the latest from Ohmeda (ignoring the desflurane-specific 'Tec 6).

➡ **It is a concentration-calibrated, flow-compensated, temperature-compensated plenum vaporiser.**

The features and benefits are:

- The fresh gas flow is divided into two on entering the vaporiser. Part flows to the vaporising chamber, and part flows through a by-pass channel. The exact ratio of the two flows is set by the dial on the top, calibrated for delivered concentration.

- Before the fresh gas flow enters the vaporising chamber it passes through a long helical pathway. This is designed to ensure that there is no chance of saturated gas passing out of the vaporisation chamber in a retrograde direction. This may occur due to the back pressure that develops during positive pressure ventilation with a gas-driven ventilator (e.g. the Manley). Gas that flows backwards out of the vaporisation chamber may then entering the by-pass channel. This is the 'pumping effect'.

- In order to ensure as close to full vaporisation as possible (i.e. vapour at saturated vapour pressure (svp)) the fresh gas flow in the vaporisation chamber is passed over a spiral wick that ensures a large surface area for vaporisation to occur.

- The fresh gas flow in the by-pass channel passes over a bimetallic strip that restricts the by-pass flow at lower temperatures, so increasing the ratio that passes into the vaporisation chamber when the svp is lower.

- The vaporiser is attached to the back bar by locating it on two pins on the Selectatec manifold. It cannot be mounted when it or any other attached vaporiser is switched on. Once located the vaporiser must be locked in position by means of a push-and-twist action on the locking lever at the back. It is impossible to switch the dial on until this has been done. This helps to ensure correct positioning of the vaporiser before it is used.

- The dial itself features a lock at the back that has to be released before it can be turned. This is easier to do than the rather stiff lock on the 'Tec 4 series. It is only when the dial release is pressed that two plungers open valves in the Selectatec manifold and so allow the fresh gas flow to pass into the vaporiser. Until this is done the vaporiser is isolated from the fresh gas flow. The dial release also activates two horizontal rods that prevent use of any other Selectatec vaporiser on the manifold.

- The vaporiser is designed so that its accuracy is not compromised by inversion or use at an angle.

- The vaporiser has a highly visible level indicator that shows the amount of liquid present, and also gives an indication of the volume required to refill it. It is able to take a larger volume of volatile agent than the 'Tec 4 series so increasing the filling interval.

- Refilling requires use of a keyed filler so reducing the risk of the incorrect agent being used. The mechanism is relatively simple and the amount of spillage during filling is considerably reduced, so both waste and atmosphere contamination is reduced (though with the latter it should be noted that the COSHH recommendations are that all vaporisers are refilled in a fume chamber). Furthermore the vaporiser cannot be overfilled.

....

4. WHAT IS THE DIFFERENCE BETWEEN A PLENUM AND A DRAW-OVER VAPORISER?

➡ **Vaporisers can be separated into two groups by considering their resistance to fresh gas flow.**

The plenum vaporiser (e.g. the 'Tec series) is a high resistance vaporiser designed for use where the driving force of the fresh gas flow is the pressure from a pipeline or cylinder supply. It is therefore of use outside the anaesthetic breathing circuit (specifically outside a circle system - VOC). The vaporiser is designed to be accurate in its calibrated delivery of vapour and in order to do this it needs to provide as near to complete vaporisation as possible. This it does within the 'plenum' chamber (meaning 'a chamber whose pressure is higher within than outside') by use of wicks, baffles or bubbling that increase the time of contact between the fresh gas flow and the liquid surface and increase the area of contact. These methods offer high resistance to the flow of the fresh gas and so can only be used where that flow can be maintained despite the resistance.

Draw-over vaporisers (e.g. the Goldman) are designed to be used in situations where there must be minimal resistance to flow. If the vaporiser is used inside a circle (VIC) the gas flow is driven by the patient's inspiratory effort. In this case it is important to keep the resistance low, and accuracy of calibration and efficiency of vaporisation are secondary to this. The Goldman vaporiser is a simple container with a variable splitting control that allows a proportion of the gas to enter the vaporisation chamber. The chamber itself consists of nothing more than a quantity of liquid over which the gas flow passes, with none of the complexities or enhancements of the plenum vaporiser.

....

5. HOW WOULD YOU ASSESS THE PRESENCE OF ISCHAEMIC HEART DISEASE PREOPERATIVELY?

➡ **Clinically, and especially from the history, in the first instance: see above.**

➡ **Chest X-ray is not useful unless failure is present.**

The electrocardiogram

This is useful, but only shows established changes and may be normal in the presence of ischaemic heart disease (IHD). However features of ischaemia include:

Features of old myocardial infarction:

- ST depression
- Q waves   } in affected leads
- T wave inversion

Features of existing ischaemia:

- ST depression, commonly laterally
- Poor R wave progression through the anterior leads

Exercise electrocardiography

- Chest pain accompanied by >2 mm ST depression is considered diagnostic of IHD
- Drop in blood pressure is suggestive of IHD

Thallium scanning

This uses injected thallium-201 which is taken up into cardiac muscle in proportion to the degree of perfusion. The isotope is detected with a gamma-camera, demonstrating perfused areas, which can be scarred or ischaemic. The distinction is made by injecting a coronary vasodilator, such as dipyridamole; if an area is reversibly ischaemic, it will dilate and light up after administration of dipyridamole. It may then be appropriate to revascularise such areas before elective surgery.

Echocardiography

1. Abnormalities of wall motion indicate ischaemia or scarring. These are:

- Hypokinesis
- Akinesis
- Dyskinesis
- Reduced systolic thickening

2. Global dysfunction indicates a more severe disorder, and is represented by:

- ↑End-diastolic dimension
- ↓Ejection fraction – which can also be detected on multiple uptake gated acquisition (MUGA) which uses technetium-99 labelled red cells. This is not a first-line investigation for IHD.

Holter 24-hour ST segment monitoring

This is an increasingly used investigation, observing as it does the pattern of ST morphology over an extended period. Holter monitoring was originally employed for the detection of arrhythmias. It has been found to be a highly significant predictor of postoperative cardiac events.

Pulmonary Artery Monitoring

While IHD causes decreased ventricular compliance, increased left ventricular end diastolic pressure and elevated wedge pressure, it is not an investigation routinely employed in this context.

••••••••••••••••••••••••••••••

6. HOW COMMON IS ISCHAEMIC HEART DISEASE AND WHAT CLINICAL FEATURES ARE SUGGESTIVE OF ITS PRESENCE?

➡ **This is not asking about investigations**

➡ **Ischaemia occurs when oxygen demand exceeds supply**

In 1982, Lunn and Mushin described the prevalence of cardiovascular disease in the general surgical population as follows:

Age 40 – 50:	6%
Age 50 – 60:	23%
Age 60 – 70:	45%
Age over 70:	100%.

It is therefore present in a high proportion of the surgical population.

History of myocardial infarction is an obvious feature, as is angina pectoris. However silent ischaemia is three times as common as angina; it occurs in the morning more than the afternoon, in the elderly, and in diabetics. Other risk factors include:

• Tobacco consumption
• Hypertension
• Obesity
• Family history
• High cholesterol – although this is becoming increasingly controversial

Other more subtle symptoms can be equally important. These include features of congestive cardiac failure:

• Coughing on lying flat
• Unexplained insomnia and nocturia
• Unexplained tachycardia or arrhythmias
• Dyspnoea accompanying angina, which is pathognemonic of transient left ventricular failure
• Chronic fatigue

Goldman identified heart failure as the single most significant risk factor for anaesthesia.

••••••••••••••••••••••••••••••

7. HOW DO YOU ESTIMATE OBESITY?

➡ **Obesity is common and increasing in the surgical population, and occurs in the female whose fat comprises more than 30% of her body weight, and in men when more than 25% of the body weight is fat.**

Ideal body weight can be calculated by subtracting 100 (men) or 105 (women) from the height in cm.

For example: height 178: ideal weight = 178 – 100 = 78 kg

There are a number of ways of estimating obesity. The commonest is the Quetelet index:

Body mass index (BMI) = weight (kg) / height (m^2).

<20	=	underweight
20 – 25	=	normal
25 – 30	=	overweight
30 – 35	=	obese
>35	=	morbidly obese

For example:

Height 1.78^2 = 3.17

Weight   = 77 kg

BMI   = 77 / 3.17 = 24; in the normal range.

For example:

Height 1.50^2 = 2.25

Weight   = 95 kg

BMI   = 95 / 2.25 = 42; morbid obesity.

••••••••••••••••••••••••••••••••

8. WHAT PROBLEMS DO YOU CONSIDER PREOPERATIVELY IF OBESITY IS PRESENT?

➡ **Organise your answer by systems**

➡ **The commonest problem in obesity is control of the airway**

Cardiovascular changes

- Increased cardiac output and cardiac work
- Hypertension (sleep hypoxaemia and increased erythropoeitin leading to polycythaemia; increased sympathetic activity; increased cardiac output; activated renin-angiotensin-aldosterone system)
- Increased stroke volume and left ventricular dimensions; this may proceed to LV failure
- Right ventricular hypertrophy and dilation, proceeding to RV failure
- Coronary artery disease (cholesterol, decreased high density lipoproteins, HDL) and ischaemic heart disease
- Cardiac arrhythmias (due to IHD, high catecholamines and increased cardiac work; fatty infiltration of cardiac muscle may also occur)

Respiratory changes

- Increased tendency to hypoxia: increased $\dot{V}O_2$ and CO_2 production, $\dot{V}/\dot{Q}$ mismatch and intrapulmonary shunt; patients also have high incidence of pulmonary disease
- Decreased pulmonary compliance, increasing the work of breathing (by 200% compared to the non-obese patient) and impairing breathing under anaesthesia
- Decreased functional residual capacity (FRC); also a shunt of 25% may be expected under GA
- Postoperative hypoxia is more common in obese patients

Gastrointestinal changes

- Gastro-oesophageal reflux (present in 75% of obese patients)
- Liver disease; fatty change and gallstones

Pharmacological changes

- Reduced fraction of total body water
- Increased adipose compartment
- Increased cardiac output
- Increased free fatty acids, triglycerides, cholesterol and α-1 acid glycoprotein

Other changes

- Difficult venous access
- Positioning: in extreme cases, may need two operating tables.

●●●●●●●●●●●●●●●●●●●●●●●●●●●●●

9. WHAT IS INDUCED HYPOTENSION?

➡ **This is the deliberate, controlled reduction of systemic blood pressure during an anaesthetic in order to reduce blood loss or to improve the surgical field**

It is employed in situations which include:

- Middle ear surgery
- Maxillofacial surgery
- Orthopaedic surgery: back surgery (improves the field), hip arthodoesis (improved cement penetration)
- Aneurysm surgery, reducing blood loss
- Plastic surgery, controlling perfusion of microvascular anastomoses

The main contraindication to the use of induced hypotension is the presence of cardiovascular disease (myocardial infarction) or cerebrovascular disease (stroke). A diseased vascular tree is incompliant and hypotension will severely diminish Cerebral Blood Flow (CBF) and myocardial filling.

Induced hypotension is most often elicited by the use of specific agents. These include:

- Labetalol: combined α and β blocker
- Glyceryl trinitrate (GTN) (or rarely, nitroprusside): vasodilators
- Trimetaphan: ganglion blocker

It may also be induced by increased depth of anaesthesia, especially with volatile anaesthetic agents and especially isoflurane, which is a vasodilator. Also, by using other drugs as part of the anaesthetic technique which are known to have hypotensive side-effects, for example opiates and non-depolarising neuromuscular blockers such as curare. These achieve their effects through histamine release, which is often undesirable, and by ganglion blockade.

A regional anaesthetic technique which induces a sympathetic block will therefore induce hypotension.

•••••••••••••••••••••••••••••••

10. WHAT ARE THE PROBLEMS WITH INDUCED HYPOTENSION?

➡ **Induced hypotension should not be used to make a difficult operation easy but it is justified if used to make the impossible, possible**

The problem is of assuring cerebral perfusion and normal postoperative psychomotor function. Intracranial pressure (ICP) is the pressure within the vault of the skull, and is normally 10 - 15 cmH_2O. Safe anaesthesia requires adequate perfusion of the brain with blood. This in turn is dependant on Cerebral Perfusion Pressure (CPP).

CPP = MAP - (ICP + CVP)

(where MAP = Mean Arterial Pressure, which is Diastolic + 0.3 Pulse Pressure)

Autoregulation is the ability of the brain (or of any tissue) to control its own blood supply - Cerebral Blood Flow, CBF - within certain limits. The cerebral arterioles constrict as the cerebral arterial pressure rises, protecting against too high a pressure, and dilate as the pressure diminishes, allowing more blood to perfuse the brain. This operates between MAP of 60 - 130 mmHg, which is why the MAP is the most useful reading (as well as the most accurate) on the Dinamap. Autoregulation, and the protection it provides, is abolished by hypoxia, hypercapnia and trauma, as well as volatiles. It may sometimes be restored by hyperventilation.

The brain uses a large amount of oxygen, about 20% of resting oxygen consumption. The brain is an obligate glucose consumer, and stores no glucose, relying entirely on supply. The energy consumption of the brain may be equated with its rate of oxygen consumption. $CMRO_2$ is the Cerebral Metabolic Requirement for Oxygen:

$CMRO_2$ = CBF x a-vDO_2

....

11. HOW MAY INDUCED HYPOTENSION BE SAFE?

➡ **By consideration of cerebral blood flow and CMRO$_2$**

Preserving CBF

1. Direct invasive arterial monitoring for beat-to-beat pressure recording.
2. Readily-available means of reversing hypotension: large-bore venous access and immediately-available vasopressor.
3. Use of short-acting and readily-reversible drugs such as GTN.
4. Maintaining Mean Arterial Pressure (MAP) above 50 mmHg if possible, lowering below this figure for short periods only.
5. Use of a vasodilator in preference to a negative inotrope, since vasodilation improves cerebral perfusion.
6. Use of high inspired oxygen fractions.
7. Posture: cerebrum lower than sternum.

Reducing CMRO$_2$

Adequate depth of anaesthesia.

Use of agents which are known to depress CMRO$_2$ such as thiopentone, propofol and isoflurane.

••••••••••••••••••••••••••••••

12. HOW DO YOU MANAGE A CASE OF ACUTE POISONING?

➡ **You must begin by discussing resuscitation**

1. Resuscitation: Airway, Breathing, Circulation.

2. Cannulation

   – and samples to lab for immediate paracetamol and salicylates, retain serum for toxicology.

3. History

   from Ambulance crew and family.

4. Empty stomach

   (not in case of paraffin ingestion – risk of aspiration) and instillation of activated charcoal (even in delayed presentation, as it may interrupt enterohepatic circulation of drugs). Leave in NG tube.

5. Secondary survey:

   Chest Xray; arterial blood gas analysis (ABG) for detection of acidosis and distinction between metabolic, and respiratory, patterns; urinary catheter.

6. Specific antidotes:

β blockers	atropine, isoprenaline, glucagon
CO	hyperbaric O_2 ($t_{1/2}$ of COHb is 250 min in air, 50 min in 100% O_2, and 22 min at 2.5 bar).
Cyanide	dicobalt edetate 20 ml i.v. chelates CN, Na thiosulphate 50 ml 25% presents sulphur substrate for enzyme.
Opioids	naloxone
Benzodiazepines	flumazenil
Paracetamol	acetylcysteine
Digoxin	Digoxin-specific Fab antibody fragments (Digibind)
Metals	chelating agents: desferrioxamine, dimercaprol, penicillamine.
Organophosphorus	atropine, oximes, pyridostigmine (prophylaxis).

7. Specific measures:

   e.g. pacing in tricyclic antidepressant toxicity.

8. Diuresis or dialysis:

   Aim to keep urinary pH > 6.5 to prevent myoglobin deposition. Mannitol is better than frusemide.

•••••••••••••••••••••••••••••••

13. YOU ARE CALLED TO CASUALTY TO SEE A PATIENT WITH BURNS. WHAT WOULD MAKE YOU SUSPECT THE PRESENCE OF AN INHALATIONAL INJURY?

➡ **Consider the direct effects of burns on the airway as well as the metabolic consequences such as carboxyhaemoglobinaemia**

➡ **Inhalational injury must be considered if there is a history of entrapment in an enclosed space, and is less likely, though not impossible, with an electrical burn. Other indicators are:**

- Facial involvement of burns
- Burnt nares, soot in nose
- Stridor, which is an indication for immediate tracheal intubation
- Evidence at laryngoscopy – a give-away

Retrospective carbon monoxide (CO) estimation. The lab co-oximeter will quantify CO levels (but, of considerable importance, the bedside oximeter will not, and cannot distinguish carboxyhaemoglobin (COHb) from oxyhaemoglobin. A patient whose haemoglobin is apparently 99% saturated according to a pulse oximeter may be dying of hypoxia). If the time of injury is known, the exposure levels of CO may be calculated from a nomogram and inhalation injury inferred if a high level is calculated. Presence of COHb is also associated with inhalation of other toxins such as cyanide produced by burning plastics.

The treatment of carboxyhaemoglobinaemia depends on displacement of the CO from the Hb molecule to which it is very tightly bound. The half-life of COHb is 250 minutes in air, 50 minutes in 100% O_2, and 22 minutes in a hyperbaric chamber at 2.5 atmospheres. Getting the patient into a chamber fast enough is another matter.

➡ **A low threshold for intubation and ventilation is recommended.**

● ●

14. HOW DO YOU CALCULATE THE AMOUNT OF FLUID NEEDED FOR RESUSCITATION IN A BURNT PATIENT?

➡ **There are several methods but familiarity is expected with only one**

The Muir and Barclay formula deals with the so-called 'shock' phase of the injury, the first 36 hours, and dictates replacement therapy, dealing with colloid (Albumin solution), and crystalloid, as well as blood. This depends on calculation of body surface burn (BSB) in percent, and body weight (BW) in kg. It must be calculated from the time of injury, not from time of admission.

1. Colloid: (BW x %BSB) / 2 = mls per block.

   Blocks at 4,4,4,6,6,12 hours post injury.

2. Crystalloid: (1.5 x BW) ml/hr.

3. Blood: 50 ml/%BSB.

To monitor progress, most would now say that a pulmonary artery catheter is essential, and that the problems of infection from lines are outweighed by the advantages of reliable data on the patient's cardiovascular status. A urinary catheter is essential. The static plasma deficit allows hour-to-hour progress to be calculated based on haematocrit, and is a useful tool. It requires a knowledge of the patient's calculated normal blood volume (BV):

To calculate blood volume:

- Adult: 7% body weight, or 70 ml/kg
- Child: 80 ml/kg
- Neonate: 90 ml/kg
- Deficit $= BV - \dfrac{(BV \times \text{normal Hct})}{\text{Observed Hct}}$

• •

15. WHAT METHODS ARE AVAILABLE FOR PAIN RELIEF IN LABOUR?

➡ **Only an overview is required here.**

Transcutaneous Electrical Nerve Stimulation (TENS)

This works by means of the gate theory and is often perfectly adequate for mothers in early and sometimes advanced labour. Electrodes are placed on dermatomes corresponding to the source of pain, in other words to the uterus, T10 - L1. Low frequency high amplitude stimulation of the Aβ fibres closes the gate.

Inhalational Methods

These operate at a cortical and thalamic level, and affect conscious level. The effect is however very transient and inhalational agents will reach the foetus. In the past this has included methoxyflurane and trichloroethylene, both now unavailable. This leaves Entonox, which is 50% nitrous oxide in oxygen. The cylinders are blue with blue and white shoulders and are available in sizes D (500 litres) F (2000 litres) and G (5000 litres). Delivery is from a demand valve operated by maternal inspiration. Only about 50% of mothers who use Entonox derive adequate analgesia, and there are two other particular problems. Firstly the use of the demand valve requires some teaching, and the parturient must be co-ordinating her inhalation with the beginning of the contraction since the analgesic effect takes 45 seconds to be maximal. Secondly, there is a tendency to hyperventilation which reduces oxygen delivery to the foetus. Isoflurane may be used for this in the future as it has modest analgesic properties.

Intramuscular Opiates

Pethidine 150 mg, with further doses of 100 mg up to three times, may be administered by Midwifery staff without a doctor's prescription. The main objection to the use of pethidine is that, once administered, it accumulates in the foetus and causes neonatal respiratory depression. Metabolites of pethidine are detectable for a prolonged period post delivery. Of all the available opiates, pethidine is probably the least effective as an analgesic. It is short acting and has atropine-like effects.

Patient-controlled intravenous analgesia (PCA) is used to good effect in some centres as an alternative to intramuscular analgesia.

Regional Analgesia

Modern thinking is that this is the safest and most effective means of providing analgesia, from the point of view of the mother and the foetus. Indeed it has considerable advantages over other forms in certain situations, e.g. pre-eclampsia, where it assists in the control of blood pressure. Also in multiple birth, where the second twin is delivered in better condition, and where intervention is anticipated, when a long labour may be made more comfortable and the hazards of general anaesthesia avoided.

There are only two situations when a regional technique absolutely must not be used. These are maternal refusal and bleeding disorder. Sepsis, hypovolaemia (and the risk of hypovolaemia), and urgency of delivery are all relative contraindications. Neither aspirin nor back surgery are contraindications.

••••••••••••••••••••••••••••••

16. WHY SHOULD PATIENTS BE ENCOURAGED TO GIVE UP SMOKING BEFORE ANAESTHESIA?

➡ **There are immediate, short-term and long-term reasons to cease smoking prior to anaesthesia.**

Smokers are more likely to desaturate in recovery, as are the passive-smoking children of smoking parents.

Immediate reasons: these relate to oxygen delivery

The half-life of carboxyhaemoglobin (COHb) is 250 minutes in room air; COHb displaces oxygen from haemoglobin, but is not detected by pulse oximetry, which reads COHb as HbO. A heavy smoker (60/day) may have a COHb of 15%, so that his or her HbO is, at best, 85%. A bedside pulse oximetry reading of 92% clearly indicates much worse hypoxia in such a case. This has obvious implications for oxygen delivery. Nicotine is a sympathetic stimulant, so there is a chance of accelerated cardiac function in the context of reduced oxygen delivery. Abstinence from smoking for 12 hours restores oxygen carriage to that of the non-smoker.

Short term reasons: these mostly relate to pulmonary function

Smokers have increased pulmonary secretions and airway sensitivity. They also have small airway narrowing and a tendency to $\dot{V}/\dot{Q}$ mismatch. They have up to a 6-fold increase in atelectasis and pneumonia compared to non-smokers, and an increased incidence of laryngo- and bronchospasm. These effects are abolished after a period of abstinence from smoking of 6–8 weeks. In addition, nicotine induces hepatic enzymes and smokers have an increased clearance of certain sedative and anaesthetic drugs.

Long term reasons: these relate to malignancy and cardiovascular function

Smokers have a tendency to thrombo-embolic disease and have increased coronary vascular resistance. Tobacco smoke contains at least 43 carcinogens. The risk of pulmonary malignancy in a reformed smoker after 7 years of abstinence falls to that of the non-smoking population.

••••••••••••••••••••••••••••••

17. WHAT IS THE DIFFERENCE BETWEEN pH-STAT AND ALPHA-STAT?

➡️ **These terms relate to the acid–base management of a patient undergoing cardiopulmonary bypass, and specifically to the solubility of carbon dioxide under hypothermic conditions.**

This is a very advanced question. You will be in prize territory if this comes up.

Hypothermia to 32°C or lower is used in cardiopulmonary bypass (CPB).

pH–stat

The solubility of carbon dioxide in blood is temperature-dependant; it becomes more soluble as the temperature decreases; one way to remember this is that it is the opposite of the solubility of sugar in tea. The same amount of carbon dioxide will exert a lower partial pressure in blood under hypothermic conditions than at normal body temperature. Carbon dioxide exerts a vasodilator effect in proportion to the local partial pressure; in the early days of cardiopulmonary bypass there were concerns that cerebral ischaemia occurred as a consequence of the reduced CO_2 tension seen in hypothermia due to the enhanced solubility of the CO_2 and the consequently lowered partial pressure exerted. The principle of pH-stat is that CO_2 is added to the oxygenator so that the partial pressure of CO_2, and the pH of the blood, remains constant, at a pCO_2 of 5.3 kPa and a pH of 7.4, respectively, as measured under hypothermic conditions.

Alpha–stat

The alpha–imidazole group on the histidine moiety of cell and blood proteins contributes to the buffering capacity of blood. The degree of buffering capacity is expressed as alpha, which is the proportion of the imidazole components which have dissociated and lost a proton. Alpha-stat observes a sample drawn from the hypothermic patient for pCO_2 and pH, but measured at 37°C; it aims to maintain a non-temperature corrected pCO_2 of 5.3 kPa and a pH of 7.4. The real pH will be higher than normal, and the real pCO_2 lower than usual. The alpha-stat system disregards the pCO_2 tension and is intended to preserve the buffering capacity, and with it, enzyme function and hence metabolic activity.

The pH–stat method has been traditional, but there is now a trend towards the alpha–stat method. The argument in favour of pH–stat is the preservation of cerebral vasodilation; the argument against invokes the risk of cerebral embolisation and steal. The argument for alpha-stat is the normalisation of enzyme function and metabolism, and the argument against concerns the risk of reduction in cerebral perfusion.

•••••••••••••••••••••••••••••

18. HOW DO YOU ASSESS THE SEVERITY OF SUBARACHNOID HAEMORRHAGE?

➡ **There are at least two systems, so you should be prepared to discuss one in detail.**

If under age 18, subarachnoid haemorrhage (SAH) will be due to bleeding from an intracranial arterio-venous malformation, unless shown otherwise; this is also the commonest cause in young people over 18. In the older person, this will be due to rupture of a Berry aneurysm in the circle of Willis. There is a postulated link between childhood chemotherapy and adult Berry aneurysm formation.

Hunt & Hess Scale:

Scale	Symptoms and signs	Mortality
I	Asymptomatic, or mild headache;	0-5%
II	Moderate/severe headache; +/- neck stiffness	2-10%
III	Drowsiness, +/- focal neurological deficit	8-15%
IV	Stupor, severe neurological deficit	60-70%
V	Moribund, deep coma	70-100%

World Federation of Neurosurgeons (WFNS) Grade:

Grade	Glasgow coma score	Neurological signs
1	15	Neurologically intact except for cranial nerve deficit
2	15	As 1 but with headache and/or neck stiffness
3a	13-14	Without focal neurological deficit
3b	13-14	With focal neurological deficit
4	8-12	With or without neurological deficit
5	3-7	Coma, with or without abnormal posturing

The *Fisher grade* relates to CT scan findings and to the presence of blood in the CSF. The more blood, the worse the outcome. The grading is as follows:

Grade	Observation of blood in CSF on CT
1	None
2	Diffuse, thin sheet
3	Thick layer or clot

••••••••••••••••••••••••••••••

19. WHAT IS THE ROLE OF CONTROL OF BLOOD PRESSURE IN THE MANAGEMENT OF SUBARACHNOID HAEMORRHAGE?

➡ **Hypotension, in order to reduce the perceived risk of rebleeding, is now an obsolete concept, and has been replaced by maintenance of supranormal blood pressure to ensure cerebral perfusion.**

The period following acute subarachnoid haemorrhage (SAH) is often complicated by cerebral arterial spasm which causes focal neurological deficit. The aim of treatment, particularly with the higher scales and grades of SAH, is to preserve cerebral perfusion and overcome arterial spasm.

$$CPP = MAP - (ICP + CVP)$$

Where CPP is cerebral perfusion pressure, MAP is mean arterial pressure, ICP is intracranial pressure and CVP is central venous pressure.

Inotropic support in SAH

In order to achieve adequate CPP, gentle inotropic support is used (generally dopamine in the range 2.5-10 µg/kg/min). In certain circumstances a pulmonary artery catheter is used to optimise MAP (and so CPP) by observation and adjustment of cardiac index (CI), body surface area-indexed systemic vascular resistance (SVRI), and pulmonary capillary wedge pressure (PCWP). The point about this, which applies to neurosurgical intensive care in general (and distinguishes it, in general, from other adult intensive care) is that the cardiovascular system is not directly affected by the disease process and is being manipulated not for the benefit of the CVS per se but for the greater benefit of the central nervous system.

Nimodipine in SAH

Nimodipine is a calcium antagonist with anti-spasmodic effects. It is used by infusion from the point of diagnosis of SAH in order to reduce cerebral vasospasm and reduce morbidity. Because it has vasodilator effects beyond the brain, there is a tendency with its use for a reduction in mean arterial pressure; this is another reason for the increasing use of inotropic support in the management of SAH.

Early surgery for acute subarachnoid haemorrhage (within 48 hours) is gaining acceptance in the UK, because of reduction in risk of rebleeding, and earlier hospital discharge; it is otherwise delayed for about a week. The aneurysm must be identified at angiography. This may take place under intubated general anaesthesia, with transportable inotropic support in higher grades of SAH, with obvious implications for the anaesthetic. Under certain circumstances an aneurysm can be embolised, by insertion of a metal coil into the aneurysm sac. Previously, vasodilators such as nitroprusside were employed to drop the BP peroperatively to permit surgery on the aneurysm to take place; this was associated with a worse outcome, and so local hypotension, with temporary clipping, has replaced it.

••••••••••••••••••••••••••••••

20. HOW CAN YOU CONFIRM THE CORRECT PLACEMENT OF AN ENDOBRONCHIAL TUBE?

➡ **Fibreoptic examination is the definitive method.**

The key is to **isolate** the upper, operative lung and to **ventilate** the dependant, lower lung. After placement, follow the sequence of tests as below:

1. Inflate tracheal cuff: you should then hear breath sounds over both lung fields.
2. Inflate bronchial cuff and deflate the tracheal cuff: you will then hear sounds only on the bronchially-intubated side.
3. Then ventilate each side separately.
4. Repeat 1-3 after patient movement or repositioning.

The surgeon will invite you to "let the lung down". To do this, assuming bronchial intubation on the dependednt side, clamp the tube leading from the tracheal lumen (red marking) and remove the bung from the top of its tube; the bronchially-intubated (blue marking) tube will now ventilate the dependant lung, and the upper lung will be isolated and should deflate. If there is a leak around the bronchial cuff, however, the upper lung may reinflate.

➡ **Use of pressure-volume and flow-volume loops displayed on a monitor during surgery will identify the secondary displacement of an endobronchial tube from its original position, because the appearance of the loops will alter with time.**

•••••••••••••••••••••••••••••••

21. WHAT ARE THE COMPLICATIONS ASSOCIATED WITH EPIDURAL ANALGESIA IN LABOUR? HOW ARE THESE COMPLICATIONS MANAGED?

➡️ **Complications may be broadly divided into early and late. As a generalisation, the early complications are common and easily managed; it is the late complications which are rarer and more serious.**

Early complications:

1. Failure, which may occur up to 4%. Resiting will be necessary.

2. Unilaterality; a one-sided block. This may be due to the catheter emerging from the paravertebral foramen rather than lying in the epidural space. This may happen up in to 15%, but is less common where opioids are used in the epidural mixture. An over-long catheter may extrude through an intervertebral foramen and any local anaesthetic introduced will tend to spill out of the epidural space. If adjustment of the length of catheter in the space does not resolve this, the catheter should be resited.

3. Dural tap. A rate of 0.5% is taken as acceptable. Young people with a dural tear are likely to develop post dural puncture headache (PDPH). The epidural blood patch is the definitive treatment for PDPH; rest and epidural infusion probably just delay onset. Some PDPH will resolve spontaneously. For this reason a blood patch should not be offered until 24 hours after the onset of the headache. The long-term risk of PDPH concerns dural traction due to the reduced volume of CSF, with the traction causing a subdural haematoma. A blood patch should therefore not be delayed beyond the 24 hour point. Avoidance of pushing in the second stage of labour makes no difference to the incidence or the severity of the PDPH.

4. Total spinal anaesthetic, where the intended epidural dose goes into the subarachnoid space. For this to happen, a large dose of local anaesthetic must be delivered, such as 15 ml of 0.5% bupivacaine; there will be progressive ascending weakness, hypotension, respiratory failure, and, with the airway protective reflexes obtunded, a risk of aspiration. Management involves early recognition and resuscitation; intubation and ventilation, elevation of the feet with uterine displacement, vasopressors, and fluids will be required. However, in epidural analgesia for labour, very low concentrations of local anaesthetic are used. It has been shown that if the total epidural top-up of 15 ml of 0.1% bupivacaine, which is intended to be given by the midwife, is instead placed in the subarachnoid space, a dense block to T4 ensues; for a total spinal to happen, the amount of bupivacaine needs to be very much greater. It is possible to cause a total spinal with the amount of bupivacaine used for epidural Caesarean section.

5. Inadvertent intravenous injection will cause cardiovascular toxicity. The cardiac collapse to central nervous system toxicity (CC/CNS) ratio dictates the relative safety of different agents; it compares the dose required to produce systemic CNS effects (oral tingling, depression of conscious level) to those levels required to produce cardiovascular effects. The CC/CNS ratio is 7:1 for lignocaine but only 3:1 for bupivacaine. The treatment of local anaesthetic-induced arrhythmia is Bretylium, 7 mg/kg.

6. Anaphylaxis: this is very rare, since preservatives, which are the usual implicated component, are not used in spinal or epidural anaesthesia.

7. Minor side effects include a degree of sympathetic block, which should be treated with vasopressors; shivering, which is lessened by the addition of an opioid to the epidural mixture, and pruritis, caused by the opioid, which may be troublesome. Pruritis may be treated by naloxone in small doses although the risk of abolishing some of the analgesic effect exists.

8. Complications due to misplacement of the epidural catheter or of the Tuohy needle. There are a number of ways of misplacing the needle or the catheter, which may result in a subarachnoid block, a total spinal, a mixed block, or a subdural block. The latter is a delayed, but dense, block of sudden onset which may spare the motor component. As can be seen, neither the aspiration test nor the test dose is either sensitive or specific.

In a study where the dura was deliberately punctured by the Tuohy needle to place a catheter for neurosurgical reasons, the mean distance from skin to epidural space was 4.5 cm. From epidural space to CSF was from 1.0 to 1.5 cm; this was reduced if rotation or aspiration were performed. The lessons are clear.

NEEDLE PLACEMENT	CATHETER PLACEMENT	ASPIRATION TEST	TEST DOSE	MAIN DOSE	DURAL TEAR	OUTCOME
Epidural	Epidural	-ve	-ve	Epidural	No	Normal epidural
Spinal	Spinal	+ve	+ve	Not given	By needle	SAB & PDPH
Epidural (but nicks dura)	Epidural	-ve	-ve	Epidural	Late tear by top-up	Epidural & unexpected PDPH
Epidural (but tears dura)	Mixed	?-ve	?-ve	Mixed	Torn by top-up	Mixed block & PDPH
Subdural	Subdural	-ve	-ve	Subdural	Never	Subdural
Subdural	Subdural	-ve	+ve	Not given	Torn by test dose	SAB & PDPH
Subdural	Subdural	-ve	-ve	SPINAL SPACE	Torn by main dose	TOTAL SPINAL & PDPH
Subdural	Spinal	+ve	+ve	Not given	Torn by catheter	SAB & PDPH

Late complications:

1. Neurological: cord compression or ischaemia. Spinal haematoma is very rare and can occur in the absence of a regional block. Inappropriate motor block, dense or prolonged, is an ominous sign. It is a neurosurgical emergency. Cord ischaemia is a complication of epidural anaesthesia in the elderly, not in the young.

2. Neurological: single nerve palsies. These are often indistinguishable from those caused by obstetric trauma. Cauda equina syndrome is a complication of spinal, not epidural, anaesthesia.

3. Sepsis.

4. Bladder dysfunction: retention of urine and bladder dystonia. This is legally indefensible.

5. Backache. This is a frequent complication, but again is due in large part to the obstetrics, to posture (lithotomy) and to motor blockade. Local discomfort from the puncture site needs to be explained beforehand to the mother and is self-limiting.

••••••••••••••••••••••••••••••

22. WHAT ARE THE INDICATIONS FOR TRACHEAL INTUBATION?

➡ **Have a system. Any one will do as long as it reminds you of all the points.**

➡ **These may be divided into protection of the upper airway, protection of the lower airway, and where paralysis is required for other reasons.**

1. Protection of the upper airway, when ENT surgeons or facial surgeons are at work in the nose and mouth. This is also known as "the shared airway".

2. Protection of the lower airway, in other words, prevention of aspiration of gastric contents where there is a full stomach, an acute abdomen, and in obstetrics. Where there is cardiovascular collapse, intubation and ventilation is usual.

3. Where muscle relaxation is required, for surgery (and ventilation also, therefore) or it is a prolonged procedure, when atalectasis might occur with prolonged spontaneous respiration.

••••••••••••••••••••••••••••••

23. YOU HAVE A ROOM IN WHICH YOU ARE ASKED TO ADMINISTER AN ANAESTHETIC. BEFORE YOU START, WHAT FIVE ITEMS MUST BE PRESENT ?

➡ **This is a clever question because it really does go back to basics and discusses the things which a candidate might take for granted.**

1. A light source which is adequately powerful and which can be focused on the patient.

2. A table upon which to place the patient which tips head-down to allow clearance of the airway and to restore a fall in blood pressure.

3. A means of delivering positive pressure ventilation; a self-inflating bag and not a Waters' bag or any other breathing system.

4. A means of providing suction.

5. A skilled assistant.

••••••••••••••••••••••••••••••

24. YOU ARE UNABLE TO VISUALISE THE LARYNX WHEN PERFORMING A RAPID SEQUENCE INTUBATION. WHAT WILL YOU DO?

➡ **This is a pass/fail question. You must have a prepared plan.**

This happens at an incidence of 1:3,000 in the general population, but rises to 1:300 in the third trimester of pregnancy. The first such drill was first described by Tunstall in connection with failed obstetric intubation, and has been modified many times since. It is also appropriate for other situations where the airway is at risk of soiling with gastric contents. Oxygenation is paramount.

The key points are:

- Get help quickly.
- Recognition: if misplacement has occurred, this is seen with a capnogram.

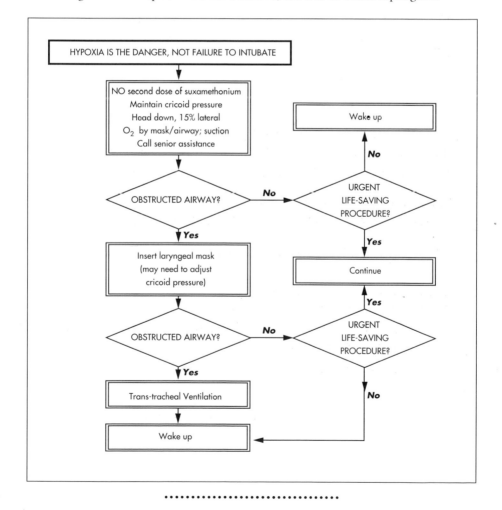

25. DO YOU SEDATE A PATIENT HAVING SPINAL ANAESTHESIA FOR HIP SURGERY?

➡ **There are valid reasons for doing so, and there are reasons not to. Be ready to present a balanced argument. There are some strong feelings in this area.**

Against:

- The choice of a regional technique may have been made in order to avoid the use of sedative drugs, so their use in addition to the selected regional technique may seem incongruous.
- Protection of airway reflexes.
- Avoidance of cardiovascular depression.

For:

- Patient comfort. Lying in one position for a prolonged period is difficult and uncomfortable. In addition, if a fracture is present, positioning for insertion of the block will be unpleasant.
- Patient co-operation. This applies to the elderly and the confused, and also to the younger patient, where a small dose of a sedative may allay anxiety prior to insertion of the block.
- Patient satisfaction. The noise of an orthopaedic saw or drill may be alarming.
- The point of using a regional block is not simply to avoid the hazards of general anaesthesia and sedation; it may also be to enhance post-operative analgesia. In this case, the arguments against may not apply.

••••••••••••••••••••••••••••••••

26. HOW DO YOU RECOGNISE, AND MANAGE, A PATIENT IN STATUS ASTHMATICUS?

➡ **This is another pass/fail question.**

Recognition:

- Often ill for several days, with attendant dehydration and exhaustion.
- Dyspnoea (inability to speak or cough are grave signs) and tachypnoea.
- Cyanosis.
- Reduced peak expiratory flow rate (PEFR) to less than 30% predicted.
- Pulsus paradoxus, especially if more than 20 mmHg.
- Arterial blood gas analysis showing reduced O_2, proceeding to hypercapnic (respiratory) acidosis.
- Beware: silent chest, drowsy patient.

Management:

- Humidified oxygen by facemask at high concentration. Young asthmatics are unlikely to be CO_2 retainers or to be dependant on a hypoxic drive to breathe.
- Bronchodilators by nebuliser or infusion.
- Hydrocortisone 4 mg/kg IV.
- Antibiotics.
- Intravenous fluids to correct dehydration.
- The question of ventilation will need to be discussed if the patient is exhausted or if CO_2 accumulating.

••••••••••••••••••••••••••••••

27. WHAT DO YOU THINK OF WHEN YOU ASSESS A PATIENT WITH RHEUMATOID ARTHRITIS?

➡ **Rheumatoid arthritis (RA) affects 3% of the population, in a ratio of 3:1 female:male. It is therefore a common condition and many affected patients present for surgery and anaesthesia.**

Rheumatoid arthritis has an insidious onset from the 4th decade of life onwards. Seropositive (IgM) RA is more common in people with HLA-DR4 than in the general population, and hence there is a genetic influence.

➡ **Divide your answer into consideration of each physiological system in turn.**

Cardiovascular considerations

10% have a pericarditis, which is often asymptomatic. 30% have a small pericardial effusion; rheumatoid nodules may form in the cardiac conducting tissues. The vasculitis may cause Raynaud's phenomenon and nailbed, cranial, coronary and mesenteric infarcts. There is a chronic anaemia (a haemoglobin of 10 g/dl is common) which correlates inversely with the erythrocyte sedimentation rate (ESR). This is worsened by the inevitable non-steroidal anti-inflammatory drug (NSAID) therapy these patients are prescribed.

Respiratory considerations

Pleural rubs, nodules and effusions are common, but rarely serious. Parenchymal disease is common if you look for it, but fibrosing alveolitis develops in only 2%, although it has a poor prognosis. RA with pneumoconiosis is Caplan's syndrome, a disease of massive confluent pulmonary rheumatoid nodules. Chest wall compliance decreases due to stiff costovertebral and intervertebral joints.

Musculoskeletal

There will be a symmetrical arthropathy involving interphalangeal joints, metacarpophalangeal joints, wrists, knees and ankles. Temporomandibular joints may be affected, reducing mouth opening, and RA affecting the cricoarytenoid joints, although described, is extremely rare. The terminal interphalangeal joint is never affected. Morning stiffness is characteristic, as is a return of symptoms in the evening – "vesperal" stiffness. Of most concern is involvement of the occipito-atlanto-axial joint (OAA), and especially of subluxation (atlas slides forward on axis) in flexion where ligamentous laxity and erosion of the odontoid peg exist. Identification of this is notoriously difficult. 25% will have radiological evidence, while only 5% will have problems. Cervical myelopathy is a serious consideration. Neck involvement is late, and affects the top end – the OAA complex – in contrast to osteoarthritis, which affects the bottom end.

Renal considerations

Amyloid deposition may occur.

Other considerations

Peptic ulceration is common. Sjögen's syndrome (keratoconjunctivitis sicca), scleritis and uveitis may be present. The patient will have been on steroids and other immunosuppressants. Gold causes marrow suppression, pulmonary fibrosis and both renal and hepatic impairment. Infections, both intra- and extra-articular, are common.

••••••••••••••••••••••••••••••

28. WHAT ARE THE PROBLEMS WITH INTRAVENOUS REGIONAL ANAESTHESIA?

➡ **Intravenous regional anaesthesia (IVRA, Bier's block) employs a large amount of local anaesthetic constrained in a limb only by a pressurised tourniquet, and is sometimes practised by non-anaesthetic doctors, for example in Accident & Emergency. These facts emphasise the hazards.**

- **The task must not be underestimated.** Full resuscitation kit must be to hand, the task should be undertaken by a doctor skilled in the technique, and the patient must be starved and full monitoring applied.
- The cuff is uncomfortable and unpleasant. The technique of inflating a lower cuff (which would then overly anaesthetised skin) and then deflating the upper cuff implies the hazard of allowing the prilocaine to enter the circulation.
- Injection of anaesthetic which is either too fast or made proximally on the limb may enter the systemic circulation. (See – *Why should you not inject into a cannula placed in the ante-cubital fossa when performing intravenous regional anaesthesia ?*)
- Local anaesthetic toxicity is a danger; bupivacaine should not be used, and prilocaine is the most popular choice, at 5 mg/kg. Prilocaine carries with it the risk of methaemoglobinaemia although it is the least cardiovascularly-toxic of the amide local anaesthetics in common use.
- A vasoconstrictor must not be used. The absence of a vasoconstrictor limits the effective duration of the block, which is not more than 90 minutes in any case.
- The quality of post-operative analgesia is poor in contrast to other regional blocks, e.g. spinal or plexus blocks.
- It cannot be used in sickle cell conditions.

••••••••••••••••••••••••••••••

29. HOW DO YOU PERFORM INDUCTION OF ANAESTHESIA FOR EPIGLOTTITIS?

➡ **Epiglottitis is caused by *Haemophilus influenzae* type B and is seen between the ages of 3 - 6 years. The adult form is rare but possible.**

➡ **Another pass/fail question. The first most important thing is to alert senior help and that of an Ear, Nose and Throat surgeon. Have a skilled assistant with you.**

1. Create a calm atmosphere; avoid moving the child, withhold cannulation or examination; do not lie the child down. Humidified oxygen, if it does not terrify the child, will help.

2. Ensure availability of emergency measures for airway control, i.e. tracheostomy. Either know how to perform a transcutaneous tracheostomy, or have an ENT surgeon to hand.

3. Perform a gaseous induction of anaesthesia, in the sitting position. Halothane in 100% oxygen remains the agent of choice, as there is no published experience of sevoflurane in this context.

4. Intubate the trachea. The laryngeal opening is where it always is, behind the epiglottis, but the only clue may be the appearance bubbles from between the cords.

5. Once the airway is secure, obtain venous access and give atropine and fluids.

6. Intravenous antibiotics: chloramphenicol or cefotaxime.

7. The child will have to remain intubated, with or without ventilation, for 24 hours. The trachea can usually be extubated uneventfully after this time if there is a leak around the tube.

   See below.

   •••••••••••••••••••••••••••••

30. WHY ARE GASES HUMIDIFIED?

Inspiring dry gases leads to a number of problems

1. Dried, tenacious secretions and mucus plugs that may physically block the airways or be difficult to clear.

2. Alveolar water evaporating to vapour increases the insensible fluid loss from the patient.

3. The evaporation of the moisture causes cooling due to the latent heat of evaporation.

4. Cilia are inhibited by dry gases and further inhibited as the airways are cooled.

5. Prolonged exposure to dry air leads to keratinisation of the epithelium and loss of the cilia.

   •••••••••••••••••••••••••••••

31. HOW ARE GASES HUMIDIFIED?

➡ **Humidification is now most easily and frequently managed by using a heat-moisture exchanger (HME).**

Methods of humidification include the following

Water droplets may be instilled directly into the trachea, however this is highly unsatisfactory as there is a risk of a condition similar to acid-aspiration syndrome.

The most common method used in theatres is the heat-moisture exchanger (or condenser humidifier). This consists of a metal or paper mesh which allows the moisture normally lost during expiration to be made available to humidify the gases on the next inspiration. In tropical conditions the temperature difference across the mesh is smaller than in more temperate conditions so there is less condensation and the HME is less efficient. The mesh can become clogged by secretions, and may be a source of infection particularly with pseudomonas.

A water bath may be used with varying levels of complexity to improve efficiency. In its simplest form the dry gases are bubbled through room temperature water, but by passing the gas through sintered glass the bubbles can be made smaller, so increasing their surface area and enhancing evaporation. If the water is then heated the absolute humidity obtainable is increased, and this can be controlled by adjusting the temperature. The operating temperature is normally 40-45°C, but as there is a large risk of bacterial contamination, the baths are often heated to up to 60°C. In this case there is a definite risk of scalding. The temperature may be thermostatically controlled by a sensor either at the bath or near to the tracheal tube. A water trap should be incorporated to remove water condensed within the tubing.

A heated element humidifier adds water as vapour to the inspired gases by dripping water onto a hot element. The high temperatures used reduce the risks of bacterial colonisation always present with water baths. These humidifiers may present problems with anaesthetic vapours as the heat may lead to decomposition.

Gas-driven nebulisers rely on the Bernoulli effect. High pressure gas flowing through an orifice causes a fall in pressure that allows entrains water. By using a baffle or anvil to divide out the larger droplets a stream of small droplets can be produced.

An ultrasonic vibrating plate (at 1-5mHz) can be used to produce the droplets, and a large amount of very fine droplets can be produced. However the efficiency of this system may lead to water overload due to uptake of large volumes of water from the terminal airways.

•••••••••••••••••••••••••••••••

32. YOU ARE INVITED TO ANAESTHETISE SOMEONE WITH A THYROID GOITRE. WHAT CONSIDERATIONS DO YOU MAKE?

➡ **You should consider the possibility of an endocrine disturbance, the risk of a deformity of the airway (per- or post operatively), and the risk of existing or operatively-induced recurrent laryngeal nerve damage.**

The presence of a goitre is consistent with hypo-, hyper-, or euthyroid function. Biochemical thyroid function testing is therefore mandatory. Thyroid disorder is covered in Volume 1. Briefly, the risks of hyperthyroidism are:

- Cardiac dysrhythmia, especially tachycardia, and atrial and ventricular fibrillation;
- Uncontrolled hypertension;
- Cardiac ischaemia;
- Excessive haemorrhage;
- Thyroid storm.

The airway must be assessed clinically and with a thoracic inlet Xray. This will reveal deviation or compression of the trachea, and allow planning of the means of airway control and anticipation of a difficult intubation; a smaller tube than usual will be needed, and elective tracheostomy has been described for massive goitre. The thoracic inlet is 10 x 5 cm and kidney-shaped, inclined 60° forwards and bounded by the first thoracic vertebra, the first ribs, and the manubrium. The trachea's integrity may be dependant upon the goitre, in which case tracheomalacia, with collapse of the trachea on inspiration, may occur postoperatively.

....

33. WHAT IS WRITTEN ON THE OUTSIDE OF A PLASTIC ENDOTRACHEAL TUBE?

➡ **You may be shown one in the viva exam.**

- Internal diameter, in mm.
- External diameter, in mm.
- Length from tip, in centimeters.
- Whether for oral or nasal use or either.
- There is a line arranged transversely above the cuff indicating the ideal position for the tube adjacent to the vocal cords.
- I.T. Z.79. I.T. refers to implant testing, and Z.79 to the Z79 Toxicity Subcomittee of the American National Standards Institute. This was set up in 1968 and establishes the current method of test. Four samples of the plastic used in the manufacture of the tube are placed in the paravertebral muscles of anaesthetised rabbits, along with reference plastic. The rabbits are sacrificed after 70 hours and the implant sites tested microscopically for evidence of inflammation.
- Manufacturer's name.

....

34. WHAT CRITERIA MAKE A PATIENT APPROPRIATE FOR DAY SURGERY?

➡ **Day surgery may account for more than 50% of elective general surgery. Divide your answer firstly into discussion of appropriate surgical procedures; thereafter, discuss medical, surgical, and social exclusions.**

There are many procedures carried out as day cases, and the number is increasing. Body wall procedures including hernia repair, varicose veins, circumcision, and removal of skin lesions; urological procedures such as cystoscopy, vasectomy and excision of epididymal cyst. Circumcision is contentious, because a caudal is the analgesic technique of choice; however, a motor block, though unlikely, would prevent the patient returning home. Gynaecological procedures include hysteroscopy and dilatation and curettage, laparoscopy (including sterilisation) and termination of pregnancy. Ear, nose and throat work, which involves a large number of children, include myringotomy and grommet insertion and polypectomy. Most dentistry has almost always been done as day cases and so does not get included here.

Medical exclusions:

- Cardiac: ischaemic heart disease, advanced hypertension, congestive cardiac failure.
- Bleeding disorders.
- Diabetes mellitus.
- Obesity with body mass index over 33, this varies from hospital to hospital.
- Muscular disease.
- Poorly controlled epilepsy.

Surgical and anaesthetic:

- Malignant hyperpyrexia susceptibility.
- Previous anaphylactic reaction to anaesthesia.
- Scoline apnoea is controversial.

Social:

- No transport, telephone or supervision for 24 hours.

•••••••••••••••••••••••••••••••

35. HOW DO YOU CLASSIFY BREATHING SYSTEMS?

➡ **You must be familiar with the Conway and Mapleson classifications.**

Conway classification

- OPEN: No exclusion of ambient air, no confinement of exhaled gases.
- SEMI-OPEN: Partial exclusion of ambient air, partial confinement of exhaled gases; an example is the Schimmelbusch mask.
- SEMI-CLOSED: Fully bounded system, with provision for gas overflow; examples include the Bain and Magill attachments.
- CLOSED: A fully bounded circuit, no overflow of exhaled gases; the only example is a circle with the expiratory valve closed down and with a minimum fresh gas flow. Low flow anaesthesia includes the definition of less than 3 l/min fresh gas flow.

Mapleson classification

This is the best way of describing a breathing attachment. These are semi-closed systems by the Conway classification. Few of them are circular, so describing them as circuits is inappropriate. In all cases, the arrow indicates the fresh gas entry and the bar indicates the adjustable pressure relief valve. Mapleson is retired professor of the Physics of Anaesthesia in Cardiff.

- MAPLESON A: The Magill attachment is the classical example of this. Excellent for spontaneous ventilation, as the anatomical dead space gas is reused. Fresh gas flows can then equal alveolar minute volume, 70 ml/kg. Not a good system for controlled ventilation. Sir Ivan Whiteside Magill died in 1986 having been instrumental in the development of laryngoscopy, intubation, founding the Association of Anaesthetists of Great Britain and Ireland, and giving his name to the Department of Anaesthetics at Westminster Hospital.

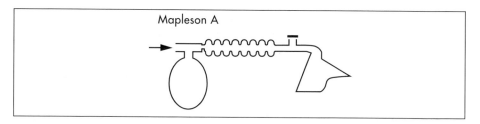

Mapleson A

- MAPLESON B: Rarely used. Inefficient.

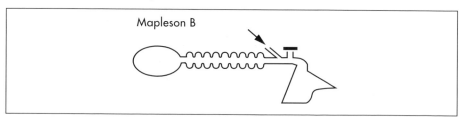

Mapleson B

- MAPLESON C: The Waters to-and-fro, used for transferring patients and for physiotherapy on the Intensive Care Unit. Originally the Waters system included a soda lime canister. Requires high fresh gas flows. Ralph Waters was the first Professor of Anaesthesia in the USA, at the University of Wisconsin. He became an academic after injuring his back in theatre and died in 1979.

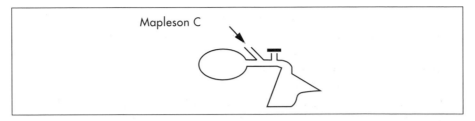

Mapleson C

- MAPLESON D: The Bain attachment is functionally a Mapleson D arrangement. This is an excellent system for controlled ventilation, requiring 70 ml/kg for normocapnoeia. Despite being inefficient for spontaneous respiration, the coaxial Bain system is one of the most popular breathing systems in the UK. Jim Bain is a Canadian anaesthetist and described this system in 1972, along with Wolfgang Spoerel; Bain's name was the first on the paper, and so it is his name which provides the eponym, and not that of his professor. Macintosh and Pask used a similar coaxial arrangement in evaluating lifejackets in volunteer subjects anaesthetised and immersed in water during the second World War. The virtue which made this arrangement useful in that context was the fact that the system could be as long as necessary; the fresh gas is delivered at the patient end, and resistance is low. This principle still applies to the Bain attachment and makes it useful in situations like X-ray and MRI imaging.

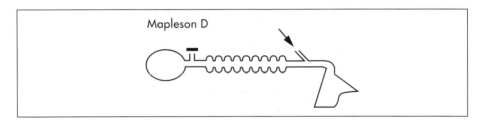

Mapleson D

- MAPLESON E: Ayre's t-piece. This is the standard system for children under 20 kg. Philip Ayre worked in Newcastle and died in 1980.

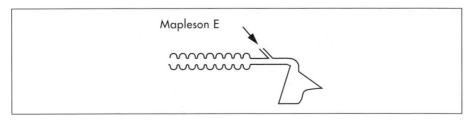

Mapleson E

- MAPLESON did not describe F, but the expression is used to describe Jackson-Rees' modification of Ayre's t-piece. This allows observation of, and control of, ventilation. A fresh gas flow of 2 - 3 x minute ventilation, and in any case more than 4 l/min. The volume of the limb must exceed tidal volume or dilution of fresh gas with room air occurs. Gordon Jackson-Rees was an anaesthetist in Liverpool.

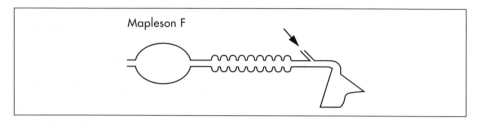

Mapleson F

. . . .

36. WHAT MUST A DAY SURGERY PATIENT DO BEFORE HE OR SHE MAY BE ALLOWED HOME?

➡ **Day surgery is growing fast and is a legitimate subject for a viva question.**

1. Adequate ventilation must be established.
2. The patient must be awake and lucid.
3. There must be stability of blood pressure and heart rate and rhythm, observed over one hour at least.
4. Swallow and cough reflexes must be restored.
5. The patient must be able to walk without fainting.
6. There must be no nausea or vomiting.
7. The patient must have passed urine.
8. The patient must have taken oral fluids.
9. The operation site should have been reviewed.
10. Postoperative instructions should have been given, verbally and in writing, and understood by the patient and the carer.
11. Postoperative analgesia must be provided. This can be simple or compound analgesics such as codydramol or coproxamol, to which may be added a non-steroidal analgesic for larger cases.
12. Proper supervision of the patient must be confirmed.

. . . .

37. WHAT HAPPENS TO INSPIRED GAS AS IT DESCENDS THE TRACHEA?

➡ **This is a question about humidification.**

Sea level atmospheric air exerts a pressure of 760 mmHg. Partial pressures are additive, and 21% of sea level air is oxygen; therefore,

21/100 x 760 = 159.6 mmHg, or 160 mmHg, of atmospheric pressure is exerted by oxygen.

However not all this oxygen is available for gas exchange, since the gas which does this is at alveolar level and differs in composition from that in the air. It is important to realise that even by taking the most colossal breath in, atmospheric air cannot be introduced into the lungs: the fluid dynamics of the airways and the moisturising effects of the respiratory mucosa see to this, by admixture with some expired gas in the first place, and by saturation with water vapour in the second.

Tracheal Inspired Gas

This has been passed over the mucosa of nasopharynx and trachea, where no gas exchange occurs but moisturisation takes place. The effect of introducing water into the air is to reduce the amount of oxygen; all partial pressures are additive, and by adding water, there is less room for the rest. The composition of tracheal gas is as follows:

- Nitrogen   76%   = 570 mmHg
- Oxygen   18%   = 143 mmHg
- Water Vapour   6%   = 47 mmHg

Alveolar gas

This is the functional level of gas exchange. However the gas in contact with the alveolar wall, and hence with the pulmonary capillary blood, is not only moisturised to the point of saturation, but also contains expired gas which contains carbon dioxide. CO_2 is extremely soluble, many times more so than oxygen, and so for most purposes alveolar PCO_2 approximates to arterial PCO_2, which is maintained in the normal state at about 40 mmHg. Alveolar gas is composed as follows;

- Nitrogen   570 mmHg
- Carbon dioxide   40 mmHg
- Oxygen   103 mmHg
- Water vapour   47 mmHg

Therefore at sea level, breathing normal air, the amount of oxygen available at alveolar level for gas exchange is just over 100 mmHg. Factors such as ventilation/perfusion inequalities and alveolar surface effects, mean that for arterial oxygen tension at sea level a figure of 97 mmHg is normal.

••••••••••••••••••••••••••••••

38. WHY DO MOUNTAINEERS USE OXYGEN AND WHY DO WE NOT NEED IT IN COMMERCIAL AIRCRAFT?

➡ **This question tests your understanding of the concept of partial pressure**

As the mountaineer climbs the atmospheric pressure falls. At sea level P_{atm} is 101 kPa, whereas at 15000 ft or 5000 m (on Mont Blanc) it has fallen to approximately 58 kPa and at 29000 ft or 9000 m (on Everest) it has fallen further to approximately 32 kPa. When air is inhaled it is mixed with water vapour which has a partial pressure equal to the saturated vapour pressure of water. This is related to the temperature in the trachea, but, assuming that this is body temperature and hence constant then this $P_{sat}H_2O$ is constant (6.26 kPa). Whilst the percentage of oxygen in the air entering the trachea does not changed (it is remains 21%) its partial pressure falls with the fall in P_{atm}:

$$P_{trachea}O_2 = (P_{atm} - P_{sat}H_2O) \times F_IO_2$$

So we now have three values for $P_{trachea}O_2$, which is also known as P_IO_2:

Altitude	P_{atm} (kPa)	$P_{sat}H_2O$ (kPa)	F_IO_2	P_IO_2 (kPa)
Sea Level	101	6.26	0.21	**19.9**
5000 m	58	6.26	0.21	**10.9**
9000 m	32	6.26	0.21	**5.4**

In the alveoli there is also CO_2 to consider as this is transferred across from the blood. Let us first consider the situation if the mountaineer does not hyperventilate, but maintains a normal P_aCO_2, and by supposition a normal P_ACO_2, of 5.3 kPa. Assuming a normal Respiratory Quotient of 0.8 then the $P_{alv}O_2$ will be:

$$P_{alv}O_2 = P_IO_2 - \frac{(P_AO_2)}{R}$$

Altitude	P_IO_2 (kPa)	P_ACO_2 (kPa)	RQ	$P_{alv}O_2$ (kPa)
Sea Level	19.9	5.3	0.8	**13.3**
5000 m	10.9	5.3	0.8	**4.2**
9000 m	5.4	5.3	0.8	**-1.2**

As can be seen our mountaineer is now severely hypoxic at 5000 m and has a negative $P_{alv}O_2$ at 9000 m, which is not compatible with life. Therefore the first thing that the mountaineer will do to correct the hypoxia is to hyperventilate and reduce his P_aCO_2 so let us now look at the same mountaineer who has reduced P_aCO_2 to 2.6 kPa:

Altitude	P_IO_2 (kPa)	P_ACO_2 (kPa)	RQ	$P_{alv}O_2$ (kPa)
Sea Level	19.9	2.6	0.8	**16.6**
5000 m	10.9	2.6	0.8	**7.7**
9000 m	5.4	2.6	0.8	**2.2**

Our mountaineer now has an improved $P_{alv}O_2$ at 5000 m, and with other more chronic compensation mechanisms (including enhanced erythropoesis leading to polycythemia, right shift of the oxyhaemoglobin dissociation curve, anatomical changes in the lungs and alteration in maximum breathing capacity) he is able to manage at 5000 m, however at 9000 m he is still in extremis, and the only way left to improve the $P_{alv}O_2$ is to increase the F_IO_2 by using oxygen:

Altitude	P_{atm} (kPa)	$P_{sat}H_2O$ (kPa)	F_IO_2	P_IO_2 (kPa)
9000 m	32	6.26	1.0	**25.7**

Altitude	P_IO_2 (kPa)	P_ACO_2 (kPa)	RQ	$P_{alv}O_2$ (kPa)
9000 m	25.7	2.6	0.8	**22.4**

This explains why mountaineers use oxygen, however in commercial aircraft to supply all the passengers with oxygen or to increase the oxygen in the cabin to allow the passengers to survive at 33000 ft would be expensive and actually carrying the oxygen would be difficult and potentially dangerous. But as the requirement is merely to increase the partial pressure of oxygen rather than the fraction of oxygen, in an enclosed space it is easier to simply increase the overall pressure to greater than that at the flying altitude. Planes are generally pressurised to the equivalent of 5-8000 ft (i.e. 80 kPa). In fact this leaves the normal healthy passenger slightly hypoxic with a saturation of around 90%, but in sick patients this could be improved further by modest supplementation (e.g. 28% ventimask):

Altitude	P_{atm} (kPa)	$P_{sat}H_2O$ (kPa)	F_IO_2	P_IO_2 (kPa)
Passenger	80	6.26	0.21	**15.5**
Patient in aircraft	80	6.26	0.28	**20.6**

Altitude	P_IO_2 (kPa)	P_ACO_2 (kPa)	RQ	$P_{alv}O_2$ (kPa)
Passenger	15.5	5.3	0.8	**8.9**
Patient in aircraft	20.6	5.3	0.8	**14.0**

••••••••••••••••••••••••••••••

39. HOW CAN THE RISK OF RECALL DURING GENERAL ANAESTHESIA BE REDUCED?

➡ **This may be divided into how you monitor the apparatus, and how you apply your pharmacological and physiological knowledge.**

Apparatus

- Check all apparatus before each operating list.
- Check ventilator, breathing system and vaporiser before each case.
- Ensure adequate servicing of equipment.
- Equipment must then be rechecked frequently throughout anaesthesia to ensure adequacy of vaporiser filling, cylinder levels, tightness of connections
- If an intravenous technique is used then the function of the pump, the continuity of the infusion tubing and the continued positioning and functioning of the indwelling cannula must be checked and rechecked.

Resuscitate

All patients should be adequately resuscitated so that adequate anaesthesia is not inhibited by the need to avoid excessive cardiovascular depression.

Dose of Induction Agent

Use an adequate dose, which may be more than the sleep dose especially in young, unpremedicated patients.

Duration of Action of Induction Agent

Ensure adequate anaesthesia is present by other means before the effect of the induction agent wears off, particularly if intubation is achieved using non-depolarising muscle relaxants that have a relatively slower speed of onset than suxamethonium.

Difficult Intubation

Between intubation attempts the patient must not only be reoxygenated but anaesthesia must be continued by inhalational or intravenous means.

Nitrous Oxide-Oxygen

This combination alone is not an anaesthetic and supplemental agents must be used.

Opioids

Conventional doses of opioid do not ensure anaesthesia, and they should be used as part of a balanced technique.

Dose of Inhalational Agents

Use of expired agent concentration monitors can help ensure that the alveolar concentration of inhalational anaesthetic agents is adequate to ensure anaesthesia.

Reversal of Muscle Relaxants

Anaesthesia either by nitrous oxide or other means must be continued until there is objective evidence of the adequacy of reversal of muscle relaxants.

Hearing

As hearing is the first sense to return some people advocate ear plugs or headphones playing music.

Amnesic Drugs

The use of benzodiazepines either pre- or intra-operatively has been suggested as an effective way to reduce conscious recall. Their use in this manner, however remains somewhat controversial.

·····························

40. WHEN MIGHT YOU SEE A VENOUS AIR EMBOLUS?

➡ **This is one of the most significant complications of neurosurgery. It occurs because veins, which are at negative pressure, are open to air during craniotomy.**

It occurs in 2 - 40% and is much more common in the sitting position, although this is rarely used in contemporary practice. The morbidity is related to the size of the embolus, which may be reduced by rapid detection. In most cases the embolus ends in the right ventricle, where it may compromise cardiac output if large enough. In cases of patent foramen ovale, a paradoxical embolus may occur with return of the embolus to vital tissue which will include the brain because of gravity.

Nitrous oxide causes any air embolus to enlarge. The use of a stethoscope and a capnograph will allow early detection, with a 'mill wheel' murmur and a decrease in end-tidal CO_2. The latter is most reliably detected with the trend display on the capnograph, as the onset of a venous air embolus may be insidious.

The management of venous air embolus is directed at stopping any further embolism by flooding the operation site with saline and packs, and supporting the circulation with 100% oxygen and fluids. Compression of the neck veins to raise venous pressure above atmospheric has been used. In some cases air may be retrieved from the right side of the heart if a central line is in place.

·····························

41. WHAT ARE THE POSSIBLE CAUSES OF HYPERTENSION IN THE RECOVERY ROOM?

➡ **The commonest cause in previously healthy patients is severe pain but other causes especially CO_2 retention should be sought before this is confirmed as the cause.**

The major causes of hypertension are all mediated via increase in the sympathetic tone.

- Pre-existing hypertension – especially if routine medication has been omitted
- Pain
- Anxiety – e. g. inadequate reversal of muscle relaxation
- Carbon dioxide retention
- Hypothermic vasoconstriction
- Hypoxia
- Pyrexia
- Drugs
  - ketamine
  - myocardial stimulants
  - vasoconstrictors
- Endocrine disease
  - thyrotoxicosis
  - pheochromocytoma
  - carcinoid syndrome
- Raised ICP
- Spinal cord trauma

••••••••••••••••••••••••••••••

42. HOW WOULD YOU MANAGE POST-OPERATIVE HYPERTENSION?

➡ **Post-operative hypertension (especially if associated with tachycardia) causes an increase in myocardial oxygen demand.**

This may lead to myocardial ischaemia, and consequent arrhythmias, infarction or ventricular failure. It also increases the risk of surgical bleeding and may put vascular suture and anastamoses at risk. In patents with raised ICP there may be a further rise in this pressure.

The actual blood pressure should be considered in the light of the patient's age, pre-operative blood pressure and co-existing pathology, though generally it should be kept below 160/100. The initial treatment is directed to correcting the causes outlined above (e.g. relieving the pain or rewarming with volume replacement). The oxygen delivery to the myocardium should be optimised with oxygen. Only if this is ineffective, and there is a risk of any of the undesirable effects noted above, then it should be treated directly, generally by use of a vasodilator.

••••••••••••••••••••••••••••••

43. WHAT ARE THE POSSIBLE CAUSES OF HYPOTENSION IN THE RECOVERY ROOM?

➡ **The commonest cause is hypovolaemia and this should be considered before other factors, though they may co-exist.**

Structure your answer according to the physiological and pharmacological factors that affect blood pressure:

Venous return (or preload)

A. Hypovolaemia
- inadequate intra-operative fluid replacement
- bleeding either overt or concealed

B. Postural changes

C. Tension pneumothorax

D. Cardiac tamponade

E. Aorto-caval compression
- pregnancy
- large intra-abdominal mass

Systemic vascular resistance

A. warming leading to vasodilation and relative hypovolaemia

B. Anaesthetic agents
- inhalational and intravenous agents
- spinal or epidural anaesthesia
- certain neuromuscular blocking agents (e.g. curare)
- opioids

C. Hypotensive agents given pre- and intra-operatively

D. Spinal cord trauma

Myocardial function

A. Arrythmias

B. Myocardial ischaemia or infarction

C. Left ventricular failure

Others

A. Cushing's syndrome

B. Myxoedema

C. Intracranial pathology

....

44. WHAT PROBLEMS DOES A PATIENT WITH SCLERODERMA PRESENT?

➡ **This is a rare condition, but appears in examinations frequently because of the anaesthetic implications. Compose your answer in a systematic fashion, dealing with the condition, then the anaesthesia.**

The disease:

- Patient: this is a disease of middle-aged women.

- Cardiovascular: cardiomyopathy and effusion are rare, in contrast to other connective tissue diseases.

- Respiratory: pulmonary fibrosis occurs late in the course of the disease but is significant, and produces a picture of restrictive lung disease. Aspiration pneumonitis is a consequence of the dysphagia and achalasia that are features of the disease. Pulmonary hypertension may occur.

- Musculoskeletal: polymyositis, which is characterised by a proximal myopathy with tenderness, running a progressive course which can come to resemble rheumatoid.

- Renal: failure of this system may be a terminal event.

- Other considerations: CREST syndrome is Calcinosis, Raynaud's, Esophageal immobility, Sclerodactyly and Telangectasia. Mouth opening is often restricted, which has implications for control of the airway when a rapid sequence intubation is required. These patients are only rarely on steroids.

Conduct of anaesthesia:

- Preoperatively: attention to the complications of the condition, as above; principally, cardiac involvement, respiratory impairment, and risk of aspiration.

- Anaesthesia: a local or regional technique is preferable, but delayed recovery of neuronal function is possible. Intubation difficulty may be expected, and with the risk of aspiration an awake fibreoptic intubation is advisable.

- Maintenance: the consideration here is the pulmonary hypertension, if present.

- Postoperatively: extubation should be undertaken remembering the risk of aspiration.

•••••••••••••••••••••••••••••

45. WHAT IS MYOTONIA DYSTROPHICA AND HOW WOULD YOU CONDUCT ANAESTHESIA IN A PATIENT WITH THE CONDITION?

➡ **This is an autosomal dominant condition affecting men and women equally, and is also known as myotonic dystrophy, myotonia atrophica, and Steinert's Disease.**

Features:

- Patient: this is a rare condition, inherited as an autosomal dominant with anticipation. There is wasting, frontal balding, diabetes, cataracts and mental retardation.
- Cardiovascular system: cardiac muscle is affected. Cardiac failure is the usual mode of death, in the sixth decade of life. Conduction defects are common.
- Respiratory system: pulmonary function is abnormal, and the CO_2 response is right-shifted.
- Musculoskeletal system: myotonia results in delayed release of contraction, as in a handshake, and is precipitated by cold, exercise, shivering, hyperkalaemia, suxamethonium (intubation may be impossible) and neostigmine.
- There are no associations with the renal system.

Conduct of anaesthesia:

- The surgery is often for cataract removal. This begs to be done under local anaesthesia. Other surgical procedures may be required, as for the general population.
- Preoperatively: 24 hour ECG may indicate rhythm instability. Lung function and ECG are mandatory. You should avoid all depressant premedication.
- Anaesthesia: Regional techniques are relatively contraindicated because of the profound weakness produced. This particularly applies to tone in the gravid uterus. Thiopentone causes profound depression, but propofol less so. Because of the likelihood of bulbar involvement, as well as respiratory muscle weakness, intubation and ventilation are essential. Suxamethonium is a disaster; atracurium, allowed to wear off at the end to avoid using neostigmine, is the preferred form of muscle relaxation.
- Maintenance: volatile anaesthetic agents cause exaggerated negative inotropic effects. Opioids also have an enhanced effect.
- Postoperatively: Intensive Care is often required, because of cardiac instability and respiratory embarrassment. The risk of aspiration is considerable.

....

46. YOU ARE ASKED TO SEE A PATIENT WITH PORPHYRIA. WHAT IS THE CONDITION, AND HOW WILL YOU CONDUCT THE ANAESTHETIC?

➡ **There are two groups of porphyria; erythropoetic and hepatic. Anaesthesia does not induce erythropoetic forms.**

The clinical effects of porphyria are due to overproduction of haem precursors, which are highly toxic, due to the overactivity of a small, readily-induced enzyme. The enzyme is δ-aminolaevulinic acid (ALA) synthetase, and the disease is due to a relative deficiency of another enzyme later on in the synthetic process, thus allowing accumulation of intermediate metabolites. The position of the deficient enzyme predicts the type of precursor to accumulate and the pattern of the disease. Smaller intermediates cross the blood–brain barrier and cause neuropsychiatric disturbance, while larger ones cause cutaneous manifestations.

The two important conditions are Acute Intermittent Porphyria (AIP) and Variegate Porphyria (VP). Both are inherited in an autosomal dominant form. Both are precipitated by induction of ALA synthetase by pregnancy, dieting, and drugs of importance such as barbiturates, steroids, sulphonamides and griseofulvin. Management of an attack involves analgesia, carbohydrate loading, β-blockade, fluids and haematin solutions to suppress ALA synthetase activity.

- Acute Intermittent Porphyria: this is due to a deficiency of uroporphyrinogen I synthase, allowing accumulation of small metabolites: thus the picture is of abdominal pain, neuropathy, and psychosis. AIP is common in Scandinavia and diagnosis is made by finding ALA in the urine.

- Variegate Porphyria: this is due to deficiency of Protoporphyrinogen oxidase, allowing accumulation of large metabolites; cutaneous manifestations of rash and necrosis occur in addition to neurological phenomena, and diagnosis is made by finding porphyrins in the stool.

Conduct of anaesthesia:

Anaesthesia: regional techniques are safe. Barbiturates are absolutely contraindicated. A safe anaesthetic includes: propofol, fentanyl, isoflurane in N_2O, atracurium, droperidol, neostigmine and atropine.

Postoperatively: adequate analgesia is essential to avoid precipitating an acute attack.

••••••••••••••••••••••••••••••

47. WHAT ARE THE DIFFERENCES BETWEEN INTENSIVE CARE, HIGH DEPENDENCY AND RECOVERY?

➡ **These are definitions which should roll off the tongue.**

- High Dependency Unit: for patients who require more intensive observation and nursing than would be expected on a general ward.
- Intensive Care Unit: for patients requiring treatment of actual or impending organ failure who may require technological support.
- Recovery Area: for patients to be admitted from an operating room, where they remain until consciousness is regained and ventilation and circulation are stable.

•••••••••••••••••••••••••••••••

48. HOW DO YOU MANAGE ACUTE DIABETIC KETOACIDOSIS?

➡ **This is a pass/fail question.**

Recognition of the condition is from a reduced conscious level, ketones on breath and in urine, dehydration in advanced cases (which may be considerable), and an acidosis with increased anion gap.

Management:

1. Resuscitation. Intubation and ventilation may be necessary, urinary catheterisation may be required.
2. Insulin by infusion.
3. Correction of hypovolaemia with saline, not dextrose, until the blood glucose is in the normal range; up to 100 ml/kg may be required in the initial phase in extreme cases.
4. Pay attention to serum potassium, which will fall with correction of glucose, and potassium supplements will be required in the infusion.
5. Bicarbonate is used only in extreme cases of acidosis.

•••••••••••••••••••••••••••••••

49. WHAT IS NCEPOD?

➡ **NCEPOD stands for the National Confidential Enquiry into Perioperative Deaths.**

NCEPOD is administered by the Royal College of Surgeons from 35-43 Lincoln's Inn Fields, London WC2A 3PN. The Enquiry depends on local reporters who are usually consultant pathologists. They report deaths, in hospital, within 30 days of a surgical procedure. A surgical procedure is defined as: "any procedure carried out by a surgeon or gynaecologist, with or without an anaesthetist, involving local, regional, or general anaesthesia or sedation." The year runs from 1 April to 31 March. 15% of reported cases are sampled, with numbered forms being sent to the consultant surgeon or gynaecologist responsible, and to the consultant anaesthetist, if identified; if not, the anaesthetic questionnaire is sent to the surgeon to be passed on. Index (or control) cases are selected by asking the surgeon to select the most recent patient for whom any of the procedures appropriate to the speciality has been performed. These patients survived for longer than 30 days.

The most recent report ran from 1st April 1992 until 31st March 1993 considering death in hospital within 30 days of surgery. This report concentrated on the 6-70 age group, and was the largest report so far, with 19816 cases. Return rate was improved in comparison to previous reports, at 72.4% of surgical and 77.4% of anaesthetic questionnaires. General recommendations included identification of a continuing shortage of HDU and ITU facilities, advocated supervision of trainees with less than 3 years experience, and recommended early conversion to open procedure at laparoscopy if problems arise. Quality of notes and lost patient records were further concerns, and the issue of "Standard of Practice", with particular reference to anaesthesia, was raised.

The key issues in anaesthesia are:

Standards of practice could be written for:
- Preoperative visiting and assessment
- Experienced staff for sick patients
- Trained non-medical staff for assistance
- Monitoring throughout cases
- Fully staffed and equipped recovery areas
- Pulse oximetry in recovery

Protocols could be developed for:
- DVT and PE prophylaxis
- Interhospital transfer of patients
- Referral of sick patients to senior staff
- Essential preoperative investigations
- Retention of staff records and duty rosters
- Out of hours operating (defined as between 18:01 and 07:59 and all day at the weekend)

••••••••••••••••••••••••••••••

50. WHAT IS IN SODA LIME AND HOW DOES IT WORK?

➡ **In order for circle systems to allow the rebreathing of exhaled gases these should be purged of carbon dioxide. This is done by absorbing the carbon dioxide with soda lime.**

Soda lime granules are composed of calcium hydroxide with small amounts of sodium hydroxide and potassium hydroxide. The latter act as activators. The other essential component is water. This is the moisture present in exhaled gases. The composition of wet soda lime is normally approximately:

Calcium hydroxide	80%
Water	15%
Sodium hydroxide	4%
Potassium hydroxide	1%
Silica & Kieseiguhr	Trace
Acid–base indicator	

The silica and kieseiguhr are added to help the hardness of the granules and minimise the formation of alkaline dust. The indicator changes colour to allow recognition of the exhaustion of the soda lime as the granules become acidotic when the activators can no longer be regenerated by the calcium hydroxide.

The absorption of the carbon dioxide involves the following reactions:

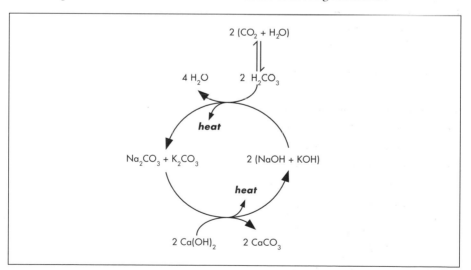

It can be summarised as:

$$CO_2 + Ca(OH)_2 \xrightarrow[\substack{H_2O \\ NaOH \\ KOH}]{} CaCO_3 + H_2O$$

• •

51. HOW COMMON IS DIABETES MELLITUS AND HOW DO YOU MANAGE IT PERIOPERATIVELY?

➡ **Diabetes mellitus (DM) affects 1% of the population but accounts for 5% of the average Trust's budget. Fifty per cent of diabetics will present for surgery during their lifetime.**

Diabetes mellitus (DM) is a multi-system disorder and has a number of implications for anaesthesia; so it is an important subject both for clinical practice and for examinations. There is a great deal of medicine in the FRCA examination, so the disease deserves thorough coverage.

The important anaesthetic considerations are:

- Vasculopathy: DM is a risk factor for an excess incidence of coronary, cerebrovascular and peripheral vascular disease. There may be obesity, hypertension, and abnormal lipids.

- Neuropathy: autonomic neuropathy is evident from abolition of beat-to-beat variation in heart rate, and abnormal response to the Valsalva manoeuvre. This predisposes to postural hypotension and extreme variations in blood pressure under anaesthesia. There will be exaggerated responses to fluid loss and fluctuations in heart rate. Responses to hypoxia and hypercarbia are unpredictable and different from the non-diabetic population. The autonomic neuropathy may also cause a gastroparesis; a rapid sequence induction is therefore advocated by some authorities. There may also be a sensory deficit.

- Nephropathy: renal failure is a common cause of death in diabetics. Some degree of renal impairment is universal, but when the disease has progressed to nodular glomerular sclerosis, it is irreversible. The picture is aggravated by the accompanying hypertension.

- Retinopathy and cataracts: these are indications for surgery.

Preoperative management:

The aim is to minimise the metabolic derangement by providing a balance of fluid, calories and insulin, with care to avoid the hazards, which are hypoglycaemia, hyperglycaemia, lipolysis, proteolysis, ketoacidosis and dehydration. The preoperative visit must establish adequacy of blood sugar control, the therapy in use, and the degree of multisystem involvement.

If you use a regional anaesthetic technique, the diabetic patient will eat sooner, have less derangement of his or her diabetic management, not be exposed to airway management problems and the risk of aspiration, will have better postoperative analgesia, and will probably be grateful.

Peroperative management of diabetes:

- Non-insulin dependant diabetics having minor surgery: transfer to short-acting agent one week preoperatively if possible. On the morning of operation, omit tablets and treat as non-diabetic if blood sugar is less than 7 mmol/l. Restart tablets with the first meal.

- Non-insulin dependant diabetics having major surgery: treat as for insulin-dependant diabetes. Once eating, convert to tds soluble insulin (e.g. actrapid) 8 - 12IU before each meal, and revert to tablets once insulin requirement is less than 20IU/day.

- Insulin-dependant diabetes: this can be managed by either the Alberti regime or by continuous dextrose and insulin by infusion. The Alberti regime involves an infusion of 500 ml 10% dextrose with 10IU actrapid and 10 mmol KCl, starting at 100 ml/hour in the adult. Blood sugar and potassium are checked every 2 hours and the infusion adjusted; this entails discarding the entire bag and starting again which is a major criticism of the regime because it is wasteful and makes accurate recording of fluid intake difficult.

- Continuous insulin and dextrose: convert to soluble insulin, and start infusion of 10% dextrose from starvation, at 100 ml/hour in the adult. Give soluble insulin by infusion; start by dividing the daily insulin requirement by 24, and giving that number of units per hour. Adjust as necessary.

·······························

52. WHAT ARE THE HAZARDS OF LAPAROSCOPY?

➡ **The laparoscopic approach used to be used almost exclusively by gynaecologists, but is now widely used by general, thoracic and even cardiac surgeons.**

These can be considered under complications of any general anaesthetic, and those specific to laparoscopy. Specific to laparoscopy are:

- Pulmonary oedema from fluid and the head-down position, which causes autotransfusion.

- The commonest structure impaled by the laparoscope is the distended stomach (1:200 - 300): so consider passing a nasogastric tube and aspirating the stomach if induction has involved prolonged manual ventilation by bag and mask. Regurgitation of gastric contents is also a risk.

- Insufflation is the most hazardous part of the procedure; 1:2000 have a demonstrable gas embolism, so beware high insufflating pressure and low flow. Signs of gas embolism are arrhythmia, hypotension, cyanosis and cardiac arrest. The safest technique involves the use of CO_2 for the pneumoperitoneum rather than N_2O, because CO_2 is more soluble and if an embolism occurs, it will resolve faster. You should watch the indicators on the insufflating machine continuously during inflation, and beware pressure over 3 kPa or total volume insufflated exceeding 5 litres. Avoid excessive head down, and always be prepared for laparotomy.

- The end-tidal CO_2 will rise during the course of a prolonged procedure and minute volume should be adjusted to compensate.

- Pneumothorax and surgical emphysema have been described, again associated with prolonged surgery.

- Caval compression and reduced venous return, with lowered cardiac output, may be a consequence of intra-abdominal pressure exceeding 4 kPa. The pressure effect of the insufflating gas will also splint the diaphragm and impede the mechanism of breathing.

- Shoulder-tip pain, from diaphragmatic irritation, is a common postoperative problem.

·····························

53. WHAT ARE THE BENEFITS OF USING A CIRCLE SYSTEM?

➡ **Although one of the commonest reasons for using low flow anaesthesia through a circle systems is economic there are a number of other reasons that are beneficial to the patient.**

Economy. It has been suggested that the direct costs of the inhalational anaesthetic agents can be reduced to less than 20% of the costs of a high flow system. This is particularly important when considering the use of the most modern agents that are very expensive (desflurane is almost universally used in the UK with a low–flow breathing system). It should be noted though that the cost of the agents themselves are only a small bart of the cost of anaesthesia and surgery, and that the costs of purchase and maintainance of the extra equipment must be considered.

Pollution. The use of low flow techniques is effective in reducing the risks of pollution in theatre and is the only way to reduce the risks to the environment by reducing significantly the total volume of volatile agents and nitrous oxide used.

Humidification. Rebreathing exhaled gases allows a build up of humidity in the inspired gases, and in a low–flow system the gases are close to 100% humidified, so the benefits of this are enjoyed by the patient (*See – Why are gases humidified?*).

Heat loss. The exothermic reaction of the soda lime heats the inspired gases, and humidification reduces heat loss further. This may be of most value in paediatric patients.

Other benefits are less obvious, but include the provision of a 5 litre sump of oxygenated gas if there is an oxygen supply failure.

•••••••••••••••••••••••••••••

54. WHAT MUST THE DAY CASE PATIENT DO, AND NOT DO, AFTER SURGERY AND ANAESTHESIA?

➡ **Instructions are given verbally and in writing to day case patients and there carers for medico–legal reasons.**

The patient must be accompanied by an adult of "suitably robust proportions", responsible for their care for first 24 hours after surgery. They must be warned, pre- and postoperatively, in verbal and written form, against driving, operating machinery, cooking, childminding, and against the ingestion of alcohol or sedative drugs other than those prescribed, for a minimum of 24 hours. One guide is that if a procedure lasts less than 30 minutes, the patient should refrain from all responsible activities for 24 hours; if the anaesthetic duration exceeds 2 hours, then the patient should rest for at least 48 hours.

Despite these instructions, there is evidence that patients disregard instructions. In one study 31% of patients went home unescorted, 9% drove home and 73% (including one bus driver) drove within 24 hours.

•••••••••••••••••••••••••••••

4 QUESTIONS ON ANATOMY

1. WHAT IS THE SENSORY INNERVATION OF THE LARYNX?

➡ **This topic often appears in the MCQ's, but also comes up in discussion on local anaesthesia for awake intubation.**

There are two watershed regions to consider when describing the sensory innervation of the larynx - the epiglottis and the 'true' vocal cords.

The superior (or anterior) surface of the epiglottis is innervated by branches of the glossopharyngeal (IX) nerve, while the inferior (or posterior) surface is innervated by the **internal laryngeal branch** of the superior laryngeal nerve - a branch of the vagus (X) nerve.

The internal laryngeal branch of the superior laryngeal nerve continues to provide sensory innervation down to the second watershed (the true vocal cords). Below the vocal cords innervation is from the **recurrent laryngeal nerve**.

The superior laryngeal nerve and the recurrent laryngeal nerve are primary branches of the vagus (X) nerve. Note that there is no inferior laryngeal nerve and that the external branch of the superior laryngeal nerve is a motor nerve to the crico-thyroid muscle.

Due to the number of nerves supplying sensory innervation to the larynx, nerve block for awake intubation is not a practical proposition. The only nerve readily (but not easily) blocked is the superior laryngeal nerve. The two most common methods of blocking the nerve are:

* application of a swab, soaked in local anaesthetic, in the piriform fossa (requires Krause's forceps).
* injection at the point where the nerve passes through the thyrohyoid membrane – either using the posterior part of the greater cornu of the hyoid as a landmark (Labat's technique) or using the most lateral aspect of the superior border of the thyroid cartilage.

••••••••••••••••••••••••••••

2. WHAT MUSCLES ACT ON THE LARYNX?

➡ **The muscles acting on the larynx have a number of actions. Try to discuss them in a logical fashion.**

The muscles in the larynx can be divided into intrinsic and extrinsic muscles.

Intrinsic muscles of the larynx

There are two distinct groups of muscles: those muscle which move the vocal cords, and those which control the aperture of the laryngeal inlet.

The muscles which move the vocal cords have attachments to the cricoid, thyroid and arytenoid cartilages. Their functions are to abduct (open), adduct (close), shorten or lengthen the vocal cords. It is vital to remember that the vocal cords attach anteriorly to the thyroid cartilage and posteriorly to the vocal process of the arytenoids. The arytenoids articulate with the cricoid cartilage. They are able to rotate or move up and down the sloping posterior border of the cricoid in response to muscular activity.

Only one muscle opens the vocal cords - the **posterior crico-arytenoid** muscle. The lateral fibres pull the arytenoids down and apart (1), while the superior fibres rotate the arytenoids (2). Both actions help to separate the vocal cords.

Two muscles act to adduct the cords (one pair of muscles and one single muscle). The **lateral crico-arytenoid** muscles rotate the arytenoids (3), while the **transverse arytenoid** muscle approximates the cartilages (4).

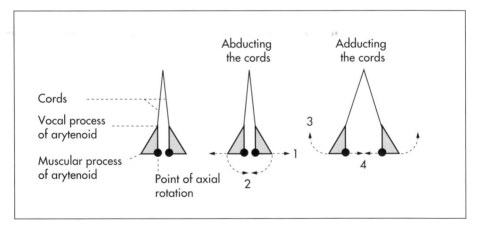

Altering the length of the vocal cords affects the pitch of the voice. The crico-thyroid muscles act to lengthen the cords, the thyro-arytenoid muscles shorten.

Control of the aperture of the inlet is provided by the ary-epiglottic and thyro-epiglottic muscles. These muscles provide a sphincteric action to minimise the risk of aspiration on swallowing.

The recurrent laryngeal nerve supplies all the intrinsic muscles of the larynx except the crico-thyroid muscle which is supplied by the external branch of the superior laryngeal nerve.

Extrinsic muscles of the larynx

The extrinsic muscles act to move the larynx upwards during swallowing and afterwards return it to the position of rest. The main elevators of the larynx are the mylo-hyoid, stylo-pharyngeus, salpingo-pharyngeus and palato-pharyngeus muscles. The depressors of the larynx are the sterno-thyroid, sterno-hyoid and omo-hyoid muscles. However, the major factor acting to return the larynx to its resting position is the elastic recoil of the trachea. The glossopharyngeal (IX) and vagus (X) nerves supply the elevators of the larynx, while the depressors are supplied by C1,2,3 via the ansa cervicalis.

Functional anatomy

All the muscles opening and closing the vocal cords are supplied by the **recurrent laryngeal nerve**.

Partial paralysis of the recurrent laryngeal nerve affects the **abductors** to a greater extent than the adductors. If one nerve is partially paralysed at operation (or by disease) the vocal cord on the same side **crosses the midline**. If both nerves are partially paralysed the vocal cords **become opposed** at the midline. While partial paralysis of one nerve causes a hoarse voice and the inability to shout and cough effectively, partial paralysis of both nerves causes severe inspiratory stridor at best and complete obstruction at worst.

If the recurrent laryngeal nerve is completely lost the vocal cord assumes a semi-abducted (or cadaveric) position. This position is seen with transection of the nerve, muscle relaxants and in death. In the living individual, this cord position is associated with stridor and vibration when air flow is substantially increased. In cases of bilateral loss the individual can only phonate in a tiny whisper.

....

3. WHAT IS THE BLOOD SUPPLY OF THE SPINAL CORD?

➡ **The blood supply to the spinal cord may be affected by surgery and anaesthesia, with disastrous consequences.**

The spinal cord is supplied by the anterior and posterior spinal arteries, reinforced with spinal branches from the deep cervical, intercostal and lumbar arteries. The anterior and posterior spinal arteries commence at the level of the foramen magnum and end when the spinal cord becomes the cauda equina. This is at the level of L1 or L2 in the adult and L3 (or even L4) in the child.

Posterior spinal artery

The posterior spinal arteries consist of one or two vessels on each side which originate from either the vertebral or posterior cerebellar arteries. They usually descend on the cord along the line of emergence of the dorsal roots. They anastomose across the dorsal midline supplying the dorsal columns (grey and white). This equates to approximately one third of the cross-sectional area of the spinal cord.

Anterior spinal artery

The anterior spinal artery is formed by the union of two arteries (one from each vertebral artery) and ends at the conus medullaris giving branches to reinforce the posterior spinal arteries. It is a midline structure running in the anterior median fissure. The anterior spinal artery supplies approximately two thirds of the cross-sectional area of the spinal cord.

The reinforcing vessels give rise to **radicular** arteries which approach the spinal cord via the ventral and dorsal nerve roots. These radicular arteries are of a variable size, but usually four to nine vessels are larger than the remainder, significantly boosting the supply from the anterior and posterior spinal arteries. Frequently one radicular artery (the **arteria radicularis magna**) is considerably larger than the rest and can be responsible for most of the blood supply of the lower two-thirds of the spinal cord. This artery is usually found in the lower thoracic or upper lumbar regions. Loss of supply from this vessel (i.e. following aortic aneurysm surgery) can lead to devastating neurological deficit, especially in areas supplied by the anterior spinal artery.

••••••••••••••••••••••••••••••

4. HOW WOULD YOU PERFORM A SPECIFIED NERVE BLOCK?

➡ **You should have a template for describing any regional technique, remembering the important points of patient explaination and consent as well as ensuring the availability of safety equipment.**

The following is good approach (though the answers to the following questions deal only with the specific points for the various blocks):

- PATIENT suitability explanation and consent.
- CANNULATE a vein.
- RESUSCITATION kit available.
- POSITION of patient.
- LANDMARKS of nerve or space, and tissues penetrated.
- NEEDLE size and length; most needles will be smaller than 22G. Pencil points are best for spinals. Short bevels cause more damage if they enter a nerve but are less likely to do so.
- ENDPOINT bone, distance, loss of resistance. The use of a nerve stimulator with an insulated needle will identify the nerve group to be blocked, as well as others to be avoided; for example, the phrenic nerve when performing an inter-scalene block.
- ASPIRATE to exclude intravascular or subarachnoid placement of needle or catheter.
- DEPTH and LENGTH of catheter for epidurals, or other situations where a catheter is used.
- INJECTION volume and concentration of local anaesthetic, with addition of opioid.
- WATCH for effects and complications, notably;
    1. Inadvertent subarachnoid or subdural injection;
    2. Inadvertent intravascular injection.

•••••••••••••••••••••••••••••••

5. STARTING AT THE EPIGLOTTIS, DESCRIBE WHAT YOU WOULD SEE DURING BRONCHOSCOPY

➡ **It is important to give distances and positions of the structures you mention.**

With the head in a neutral position, the distance from the lips to the epiglottis (in the adult) is approximately 13 - 14 cm. If bronchoscopy is being carried out by the nasal route, a further 4 - 5 cm must be added.

The epiglottis is seen anteriorly with the laryngeal inlet behind. Lateral to the epiglottis are the ary-epiglottic folds containing the cuneiform and corniculate cartilages in their upper borders. In the distance, the arytenoid cartilages are seen posteriorly with the true cords passing from their vocal process to the posterior aspect of the thyroid cartilage.

Moving distally, the vestibule of the larynx is entered. This describes the region between the laryngeal inlet and the level of the vestibular folds (false cords). The walls of the vestibule are; the inferior surface of the epiglottis anteriorly, the ary-epiglottic folds laterally and the mucous membrane connecting the arytenoid cartilages posteriorly. The gap between the false cords is called the rima vestibuli.

Beyond the rima vestibuli, the sinus of the larynx can be seen on each lateral wall, representing the opening to the saccule of the larynx.

The gap between the true cords (the rima glottidis) is approached, followed immediately by the ring-shaped cricoid cartilage. The cricoid is passed at a distance of 16 - 18 cm from the lips (at the level of C6).

There are usually 16 - 20 tracheal rings before the carina. In the adult, the trachea is approximately 10 - 12 cm long. The carina is therefore reached at approximately 26 - 30 cm from the lips. The tracheal cartilages have a posterior deficit which is filled by the trachealis muscle.

The right main bronchus branches at 25° to the vertical in the adult (45° in the child). The following bronchi are seen (distances are measured from the carina, bronchopulmonary segments are in brackets):

Upper lobe bronchus	2.5 cm at 3 o'clock	(apical, anterior, posterior)
Middle lobe bronchus	4.0 cm at 12 o'clock	(medial, lateral)
Lower lobe bronchus	4.5 cm at 6 o'clock	(apical, anterior, posterior, medial, lateral)

The left main bronchus branches at 45° to the vertical in both adult and child. The following bronchi are seen:

Upper lobe bronchus	5.0 cm at 9 o'clock	(apical, anterior, posterior)
Lingular lobe bronchus	5.5 cm at 3 o'clock	(superior, inferior)
Lower lobe bronchus	5.0 cm at 3 o'clock	(apical, anterior, posterior, medial, lateral)
Apical segment of LLB	6.0 cm at 6 o'clock	

The lingular lobe bronchus branches from the upper lobe bronchus. The lingular lobe is therefore part of the left upper lobe.

••••••••••••••••••••••••••••••

6. WHAT IS THE CIRCLE OF WILLIS?

➡ **The circle of Willis is formed from the paired internal carotid and vertebral arteries. Pressure and volume of blood flow on the two sides are equalised by the circle, but if one carotid is blocked suddenly, the anastomotic channels are usually inadequate to prevent hemiplegia.**

Having entered the cranial vault via the carotid foramen, the internal carotid arteries emerge from the roof of the cavernous sinus and divide into three main branches:

* anterior cerebral artery
* middle cerebral artery
* posterior communicating artery

Minor (but functionally vital) branches to deeper structures are also given off i.e. the internal capsule and caudate nucleus. The anterior cerebral arteries are joined by an anastomotic channel, the anterior communicating artery.

The vertebral arteries enter the cranial vault via the foramen magnum. Before they join to form the basilar artery, each gives off two branches:

* anterior spinal artery
* posterior inferior cerebellar artery

Formed at the inferior border of the pons, the basilar artery has the following branches:

* anterior inferior cerebellar artery
* labyrinthine and pontine arteries
* superior cerebellar artery
* posterior cerebral artery

The posterior communicating artery usually anastomoses with the posterior cerebral artery to complete the anastomotic circle.

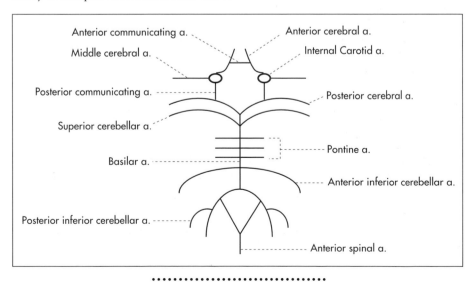

7. WHAT IS THE ARTERIAL SUPPLY OF THE HEART?

➡ **The site of a sudden coronary occlusion determines the clinical effect. Knowledge of the coronary circulation allows prediction of the likely events.**

The right and left coronary arteries arise behind the pulmonary trunk from the anterior and left posterior aortic sinuses of the ascending aorta. Anastomoses between the coronary vessels are of little functional value in the event of sudden occlusion. However, when occlusion occurs as a gradual process, anastomotic channels improve significantly.

Right coronary artery

From the anterior aortic sinus, the right coronary artery passes forwards between the right atrial appendage and the pulmonary trunk. Having crossed the infundibulum of the right ventricle, it runs in the anterior atrioventricular groove. As it travels in the groove, it gives branches to the atrium and ventricle (**atrial and ventricular short branches**). At the inferior border of the heart, the **marginal artery** runs along the right ventricle towards the apex. On the inferior surface, the **inferior** interventricular artery is given off and runs in the groove of the same name. The terminal part of the right coronary anastomoses to a varying degree with the circumflex branch of the left coronary artery. In approximately 10% of cases the inferior interventricular artery arises from the left coronary artery.

Left coronary artery

Arising from the left posterior aortic sinus, the left coronary artery passes between the left atrial appendage and the pulmonary trunk. Within a few centimetres, the main trunk divides into the **anterior interventricular artery** (or left anterior descending artery) and the **circumflex artery**. The former runs to the left in the interventricular groove, giving off a variable number of **anterior ventricular arteries**. Frequently, one of these arteries is larger than the others and is then known as the **left diagonal artery.** The branches of the circumflex artery (which continues to run in the atrioventricular groove) are inconsistent; in 90% of cases it gives off the **left ('obtuse') marginal artery**, in 35% the **artery to the sinoatrial node** and in 20% the **artery to the atrioventricular node**. It also gives off a variable number of anterior and posterior ventricular branches.

Regional supply

Right ventricle – branches of the right coronary, except for the upper, anterior border.

Left ventricle – branches of the left coronary, except for a small diaphragmatic area.

Interventricular septum – approximately equal distribution between the left and right coronaries.

Atria – variable supply, but usually from the 'same side'.

Sinoatrial node – 65% of cases from the right coronary, 35% from the left.

Atrioventricular node – 80% of cases from the right coronary, 20% from the left.

The supply of the conducting system is equivalent to the atrioventricular node.

....

8. DESCRIBE THE FORMATION AND MAJOR BRANCHES OF THE BRACHIAL PLEXUS

➡ **You should also be able to describe the interscalene, subclavian perivascular and axillary approaches to brachial plexus blockade.**

The brachial plexus is formed from the anterior primary rami of C5,6,7,8 and T1. From these 5 roots are derived:

- 3 trunks
- 6 divisions
- 3 cords
- 17 nerve branches

Roots

These emerge between the scalenus anterior and medius muscles, above the subclavian artery. Three nerves arise from the roots:

- Dorsal scapular nerve   C5
- Long thoracic nerve   C5,6,7
- Nerve to subclavius   C5,6

Trunks

The trunks are found in the posterior triangle of the neck. The roots of C5 and 6 join to form the upper trunk, C7 continues as the middle trunk and C8 and T1 join to form the lower trunk. The upper and middle trunks lie above the subclavian artery, the lower trunk behind the artery. Only one nerve arises from the trunks:

- Suprascapular nerve   C 5,6 (from the upper trunk)

Divisions

At the lateral edge of the 1st rib, each trunk gives an anterior and posterior division which pass behind and below the clavicle. There are no nerves from the divisions.

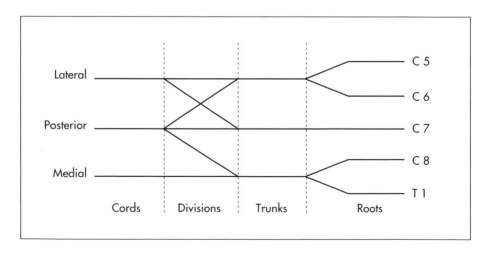

Cords

The cords are formed by the coming together of the relevant anterior and posterior divisions. The names of the cords describe their relation to the axillary artery (posterior, lateral and medial). The axillary artery, the continuation of the subclavian artery, begins at the lateral border of the 1st rib and is divided into three parts by pectoralis minor (1st part proximal, 2nd part behind and 3rd part distal to the muscle). The cords lie above the 1st part of the axillary artery, embrace the 2nd part and give branches at the 3rd part. The branches from the three cords are as follows:

Lateral cord (3 nerves)

- Lateral pectoral nerve   (C 5,6,7)
- Musculocutaneous nerve   (C 5,6,7)
- Lateral head of median n.   (C 5,6,7)

Posterior cord (5 nerves)

- Radial nerve   (C 5,6,7,8,T1)
- Axillary nerve   (C 5,6)
- Thoracodorsal nerve   (C 6,7,8)
- Upper subscapular nerve   (C 5,6)
- Lower subscapular nerve   (C 5,6)

Medial cord (5 nerves)

- Ulnar nerve   (C 7,8,T1)
- Medial head of median nerve   (C 8,T1)
- Medial cutaneous nerve of arm   (C 8,T1)
- Medial cutaneous nerve of forearm   (C 8,T1)
- Medial pectoral nerve   (C 8,T1)

••••••••••••••••••••••••••••••

9. WHAT ARE THE SURFACE MARKINGS OF THE PLEURA AND LUNGS?

➡ **This is important for both clinical assessment and X-ray interpretation.**

The pleura can be divided into parietal pleura, which lines the costal walls of the thorax, and visceral pleura, which is closely applied to the lungs.

Surface markings of the (parietal) pleura

The parietal pleura projects approximately 2.5 cm above the medial third of the clavicle.

Below the clavicle, the levels to remember are **2, 4, 6, 8, 10, 12:**

- 2nd rib — pleura meet in the midline (level of angle of Louis).
- 4th costal cartilage — right continues vertically, left arches to lateral border of the sternum.
- 6th costal cartilage — each turn laterally.
- 8th rib — cross mid–clavicular line.
- 10th rib — cross mid–axillary line and then pass horizontally.
- 12th rib — crosses the rib at the sacro–spinalis muscle (posteriorly) and reaches the lateral border of the 12th thoracic vertebra.

The parietal pleura passes outside the confines of the thoracic cage at two points:

- above the medial third of the clavicle.
- below the 12th rib in the costo–vertebral angle.

Surface markings of the lungs

The lungs also project above the medial part of the clavicle.

On the **right**, the lung markings coincide with those of the pleura down to the 6th costal cartilage. From here it passes to the 8th rib by the mid-axillary line. It then crosses horizontally to the 10th rib at the sacro-spinalis muscle and onto the lateral edge of the vertebral body of T10.

On the **left**, the heart displaces the lung to a greater extent than the pleura. The lung curves from the lateral border of the sternum at the 4th costal cartilage to the 5th intercostal space just medial to the mid-clavicular line. It then passes to the 6th rib at the midclavicular line and the 8th rib at the mid-axillary line. The remainder of the course is as for the right lung.

The inferior three markings of the lungs are seen to lie two ribs higher than the pleura (at 6, 8, 10).

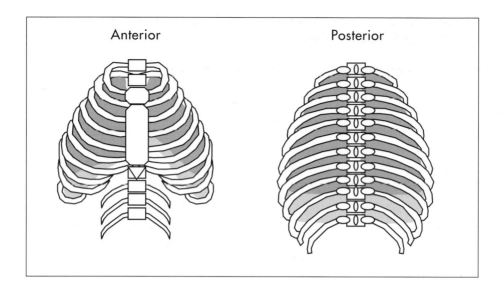

In the diagram above, the pleura is shown in light grey, the lung in dark grey.

Surface marking of the oblique fissure

- Line of the 5th rib.

  (or)

- Line joining the spinous process of T3 to the 6th rib in the midclavicular line.
  (or)

- Line marked by the vertebral border of the scapula with the arm fully abducted.

Surface marking of the horizontal fissure (right side only)

- Line continued horizontally from the 4th costal cartilage, meeting the oblique fissure in the midaxillary line.

●●●●●●●●●●●●●●●●●●●●●●●●●●●●●●●

10. DESCRIBE THE ANATOMY OF THE INTERNAL JUGULAR VEIN

➡ **You will be expected to describe how you would perform central venous cannulation (internal jugular and subclavian veins) and list the common complications of the procedure.**

The sigmoid sinus collects blood from the vast majority of the brain. Just before it exits the jugular foramen (on the inferior aspect of the skull), it expands into the jugular bulb. The internal jugular vein is the direct continuation from the jugular bulb and runs in the posterior compartment through the foramen. The position of the vein relative to the carotid artery changes during its course. Initially, it lies posterior to the artery on the lateral mass of the atlas (C1). Passing caudad, it lies first lateral and then anterolateral to the artery. Throughout their course, the artery and vein lie within the carotid sheath, with the vagus nerve between the vessels.

From the base of the skull, the internal jugular vein follows a relatively straight line, joining the subclavian vein behind the sterno-clavicular joint. In the lower part of its course, the vein is overlaid by the sterno-mastoid muscle. The terminal part of the vein lies between the sternal and clavicular heads of the muscle.

Relations of the internal jugular vein

- It lies anterior to:
  - Lateral mass of the atlas (C1).
  - Prevertebral fascia and muscles.
  - Cervical transverse process.
  - Sympathetic chain.
  - Subclavian artery, dome of the pleura, phrenic and vagus nerves(at the root of neck)
  - Thoracic duct (on the left)

- It lies lateral to:
  - Internal and common carotid arteries.
  - Glossopharyngeal, vagus, accessory and hypoglossal nerves.

- It lies posterior to:
  - Internal carotid artery and vagus nerve (on exiting the jugular foramen).

- In the neck the internal jugular vein is covered by:
- Skin and subcutaneous tissue.
- Platysma.
- Sterno-mastoid muscle.
- Fascia of the carotid sheath (relatively loose over the vein to allow expansion).

The tributaries of the internal jugular vein are:

- Inferior petrosal sinus.
- Veins from the pharyngeal plexus.
- Common facial vein (formed from the anterior facial and retromandibular veins).
- Lingual vein.
- Superior and middle thyroid veins.

The external jugular vein empties into the subclavian vein and **not** into the internal jugular vein.

•••••••••••••••••••••••••••••••

11. HOW WOULD YOU PERFORM AN ANKLE BLOCK?

➡ **Local anaesthetic blocks should only be carried out on a fully assessed, prepared and consented patient. They should be performed in an area with full resuscitation equipment, with the patient on a tipping trolley and with intravenous assess already established.**

To anaesthetise the foot at the level of the ankle, it is necessary to block five nerves:

- **tibial nerve** – at the midpoint between the medial malleolus and the calcaneus, just posterior to the pulsation of the posterior tibial artery. Via its medial and lateral plantar branches (equivalent to the median and ulnar nerves respectively in the hand), it innervates the skin and muscles of the plantar aspect of the foot.

- **deep peroneal nerve** – at the distal end of the tibia, between the tendons of extensor hallucis longus (medially) and extensor digitorum longus (laterally) the nerve lies just lateral to the anterior tibial artery. It innervates the extensor hallucis brevis muscle and the small area of skin between the 1st and 2nd toes on the dorsum of the foot.

- **superficial peroneal nerve** – at the level of the malleoli, the nerve lies in the superficial fascia and divides into a number of branches innervating the toes and dorsum of the foot not supplied by the deep peroneal and sural nerves.

- **sural nerve** – just behind the lateral malleolus, the nerve lies in the superficial fascia (in close proximity to the small saphenous vein) and innervates the lateral border of the foot and little toe.

- **saphenous nerve** – just in front of the medial malleolus, the nerve lies in the superficial fascia (in close proximity to the great saphenous vein) and innervates the medial border of the foot.

  The saphenous nerve is a branch of the femoral nerve (the only branch which passes below the knee). The other four nerves are branches of the sciatic nerve. Adequate anaesthesia is achieved with 5 ml of local anaesthetic solution at each of the above sites.

•••••••••••••••••••••••••••••••

12. DESCRIBE THE ANATOMY OF THE STELLATE GANGLION

➡ **This will usually be followed by questions related to stellate ganglion block, with a special interest in the desired effects and undesired complications of the procedure.**

The stellate (or cervicothoracic) ganglion is part of the sympathetic chain. While it is usually formed from the fusion of the C7, C8 and T1 segmental ganglia, the second (and even the third and fourth) thoracic ganglion may be incorporated. The stellate ganglion provides sympathetic innervation to the face, head, neck and upper extremity. The fusion of the C7 and C8 ganglia alone is normally termed the inferior cervical ganglion.

The stellate ganglion lies:

- Approximately level with the cricoid cartilage (C6 vertebra).
- Anterior to   – transverse process of C7.
                       – neck of the first rib.
                       – prevertebral fascia.
- Posteromedial to   – vertebral artery and vein.
                       – carotid sheath.
- Superior to   – cervical pleura (separated by the suprapleural membrane).

If the ganglion is particularly low, it may be covered by the dome of the cervical pleura.

A standard technique for stellate ganglion blockade would be:

- Supine patient.
- Head extended on the neck and looking straight ahead.
- Point of insertion 3 cm above and 2 cm lateral to the sternal notch (equates to the level of the cricoid).
- Medial to the carotid artery, lateral to the trachea.
- Insert 21G, 4 cm ('blue') needle at 90° to the skin until the tip rests on the transverse process of C6.
- Withdraw the needle 2 - 3 mm, **aspirate** and inject a test dose of 1 ml of local anaesthetic solution.
- Presuming no untoward effect from the test dose, inject a further 7 - 9 ml of solution **slowly** with regular aspiration.

Lignocaine 1%, bupivacaine 0.5% or mixtures of the two solutions are all suitable for stellate ganglion block. It is not normal practise to inject neurolytic agents around the stellate ganglion. If permanent obliteration is desired, surgical excision of the ganglia is recommended.

The signs of a successful block are ipsilateral:

- Drooping of the upper lid (ptosis).
- Pupillary constriction (miosis).
- Reduced sweating (anhydrosis).
- Retraction of the eyeball (enophthalmos).
- Venous dilatation leading to conjunctival engorgement and nasal congestion (Guttmann's sign)
- Increased skin temperature.
- Increased lacrimation.

The combination of ptosis, miosis, anhydrosis and enophthalmos is known as Horner's syndrome.

The potential complications of a stellate ganglion block are:

- Systemic toxicity (almost immediate effect if injected into the vertebral arteries).
- Vaso-vagal reactions.
- Brachial plexus block.
- Pneumothorax (approximately 1% of cases, especially in the tall, thin patients with high apical pleura).
- Recurrent laryngeal nerve block (causes temporary hoarseness).
- Phrenic nerve block (causing hemidiaphragmatic paralysis).
- Vagus nerve block (tachycardia may ensue).
- Bradycardia (due to blockade of the cardiac accelerator nerves – especially on the right side).
- Subarachnoid injection (if injected into a 'dural sleeve').

Due to the nature of the complications listed above, it is clearly unwise to perform bilateral stellate ganglion blocks at a single sitting.

•••••••••••••••••••••••••••••••••

13. HOW WOULD YOU PERFORM A PENILE BLOCK?

➡ **Be prepared to discuss the advantages and disadvantages of the block in comparison to a caudal block.**

The somatic (sensory) innervation of the penis comes from two pairs of nerves:

- Dorsal nerve of the penis – a terminal branch of the pudendal nerve (S2,3,4) which innervates all but the base of the penis. The nerve runs along the margin of the inferior pubic ramus and passes between the layers of the suspensory ligament of the penis. The nerve lies deep to the fascia of the penis (a continuation of Scarpa's fascia from the lower abdominal wall) and just lateral to the dorsal artery.
- Genito-femoral nerve – the genital segment of the nerve (L2) runs superficial to the fascia of the penis and innervates the area around the base.

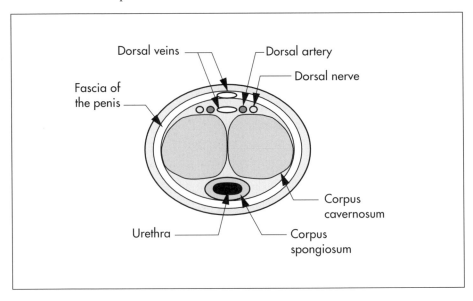

A standard technique for a penile block would be:

- Patient supine.
- Finger placed under the pubic symphysis.
- 21G, 4 cm ('blue') needle inserted in the midline, missing the dorsal vein.
- The needle is positioned on the superior surface of each corpora cavernosa (3 - 4 cm deep in the adult).
- Aspirate and deposit 5 - 10 ml of local anaesthetic (in the adult).
- Aspirate regularly during the injection.
- A further 5 - 10 ml as a subcutaneous 'ring' is used for operations on the base of the penis.

Suitable local anaesthetic solutions are 0.25 to 0.5% plain bupivacaine. The use of adrenaline containing solutions is **absolutely contraindicated** in this area.

Advantages of the penile block over a caudal:

- Easier and quicker (no need to reposition the patient).
- No motor block.
- No bladder sphincter dysfunction.
- No central sympathetic blockade.

Disadvantages:

- Erection may still occur.
- Local vascular engorgement and haematoma possible.
- Danger of intravascular injection is greater (the area is highly vascular).

••••••••••••••••••••••••••••••

14. WHY IS IT BEST TO PERFORM INTERCOSTAL NERVE BLOCKS BEHIND THE MID-AXILLARY LINE?

➡ **This question is all about applied anatomy.**

Intercostal nerve blocks may be used for abdominal and thoracic surgery, for analgesia following chest trauma and for neurolytic blocks in chronic pain conditions.

The Neurovascular Bundle

The neurovascular bundle contains the intercostal nerve, artery and vein. It lies in the subcostal groove, hidden by the sharp lower border of the rib. The bundle is deep to both the external and internal intercostal muscles. It also lies deep to the intercostal membrane. Within the bundle, the vein lies superior, the artery in the middle and the nerve inferior (VAN from superior to inferior).

Anatomy of the intercostal nerve

The intercostal nerves are derived from the anterior primary rami of the twelve thoracic nerves. They are mixed spinal nerves, containing both sensory and motor fibres. The nerves provide segmental supply to the thoracic and abdominal regions. They also innervate small areas of skin over the upper limb (T1 and 2) and buttock (T12). On the abdominal wall, the intercostal nerves (T7 to T12) run in the plane between the transversus abdominis and external oblique muscles. They then pierce the rectus sheath and innervate the rectus abdominis muscle and anterior abdominal wall.

The intercostal nerves have three branches:

- Collateral branch
- Lateral Cutaneous branch
- Anterior Terminal branch

Although the collateral branch is given off before the angle of the rib, it accompanies (and may rejoin) the main trunk in the subcostal groove. It supplies the muscles, parietal pleura and periosteum of the space. It does not normally supply any skin. The lateral cutaneous branch pierces the intercostal muscles in the mid-axillary line and divides into anterior and posterior branches. It provides sensory innervation to the vast majority of skin over the intercostal space. The lateral cutaneous branch of the second intercostal nerve is also known as the intercostobrachial nerve. It supplies a small area of skin on the medial aspect of the upper arm. The anterior terminal branch innervates skin over the anterior aspect of the chest and abdomen. It can be blocked separately with a rectus sheath block.

An intercostal block performed behind the mid-axillary line will anaesthetise all the branches of the intercostal nerve, thus achieving best analgesia.

•••••••••••••••••••••••••••••••

15. HOW WOULD YOU PERFORM A FEMORAL NERVE BLOCK?

➡ **The 'Three-in-One' technique blocks the femoral nerve, obturator nerve and the lateral cutaneous nerve of the thigh. The only differences from a standard femoral nerve block are the use of a larger volume of local anaesthetic and the application of distal pressure.**

The femoral nerve (L2,3,4) runs deep to the iliopsoas fascia on the posterolateral wall of the pelvis. It passes under the inguinal ligament and enters the upper anterior thigh. The nerve lies lateral to the femoral artery, which in turn lies lateral to the femoral vein (NAV from lateral to medial). The femoral sheath (a prolongation of the extraperitoneal fascia) contains the artery and vein, but not the more deeply placed femoral nerve. The femoral nerve divides into:

• motor branches which innervate the muscles of the front of the thigh.

• sensory branches which innervate:

- the anterior segment of the thigh (medial and intermediate cutaneous nerves of the thigh).

- the medial side of the leg and foot (saphenous nerve).

- the hip and knee joints.

The lateral cutaneous nerve of the thigh (L2,3) and obturator nerve (L2,3,4) lie in the same fascial plane as the femoral nerve on the pelvic wall. The lateral cutaneous nerve of the thigh perforates the inguinal ligament near the anterior inferior iliac spine and innervates an area of skin over the lateral aspect of the thigh. The obturator nerve (the nerve of the adductor compartment) follows a complex course in the pelvis. It supplies a number of muscles and gives sensory innervation to the medial aspect of the thigh, as well as the hip and knee joints.

A standard technique for femoral nerve block is:

• Patient supine.
• Line drawn between the anterior superior iliac spine and the pubic tubercle (inguinal ligament).
• Palpate the femoral artery at the mid-point of the ligament.
• Insert the needle at a point 1 - 2 cm lateral to the artery just below the inguinal ligament.
• Angle the needle superiorly (45°).
• Pass deep to the fascia lata (usually feel a 'click').
• Paraesthesiae elicited (or patellar movement, if using a nerve stimulator) within 3 - 4 cm.
• Aspirate and inject slowly with regular aspiration.
• If performing a 'Three-in-One' block, apply distal pressure before injecting.

Femoral nerve block alone can be performed with 10 - 15 ml of local anaesthetic solution. The 'Three-in-One' block requires 25 - 30 ml for good results.

••••••••••••••••••••••••••••••••

16. WHAT ARE THE COMMON APPROACHES FOR SCIATIC NERVE BLOCK?

➡ **Try not to forget the popliteal fossa technique.**

The sciatic nerve is the largest nerve in the body. The tibial part of the nerve is formed from the anterior divisions of L4,5,S1,2,3, while the common peroneal part is formed from the posterior divisions of L4,5,S1,2. The two parts of the nerve usually join within the pelvis to form one nerve trunk. However, they may remain separate throughout their course. Having formed at the lower border of the piriformis muscle, the sciatic nerve passes posteriorly through the greater sciatic foramen. Lying initially posterior to the acetabulum, it then passes distally over the short rotators of the hip covered by gluteus maximus. From a point midway between the greater trochanter and the ischial tuberosity, the nerve passes vertically downwards into the hamstring compartment. It re-emerges and usually divides at the upper border of the popliteal fossa. In the early part of its course, the posterior cutaneous nerve of the thigh (S1,2,3) runs on the posterior surface of the sciatic nerve.

The sciatic nerve supplies:

- The muscles of the hamstring compartment (via its main trunk).
- The flexor part of the leg and plantar aspect of the foot (via the tibial component).
- The extensor and peroneal compartments of the leg and the dorsum of the foot (via the common peroneal component).
- The hip and knee joints.

The common techniques to block the sciatic nerve are the posterior approach (of Labat), the anterior approach (of Beck) and the popliteal fossa approach. The supine block (of Raj) and the lateral approach (of Ichiyanagi) are not described.

Posterior approach

- Patient lying in the lateral position, with the side to be blocked uppermost.
- Upper leg bent to 90° at both hip and knee (lower leg straight).
- Line drawn from the greater trochanter to the posterior superior iliac spine.
- Mid-point of the line, drop a perpendicular for 5 cm (= point of insertion).
- A line from the greater trochanter to the coccyx intercepts the same point.
- 22G, 9 cm short-bevel needle inserted perpendicular to the skin.
- Paraesthesiae elicited below the knee (or muscle twitches if using a nerve stimulator).
- nerve usually found at a depth of approximately 6 cm.
- Aspirate and inject 20 ml of local anaesthetic slowly with regular aspiration.

Anterior approach

- Patient lying supine.
- First line drawn from the anterior superior iliac spine to the pubic tubercle.
- Draw a parallel line from the greater trochanter.
- Drop a perpendicular from the junction of the middle and medial thirds of the first line.
- The point at which the perpendicular intercepts the second line is the point of needle insertion.
- 20G, 12.5 cm short-bevel needle inserted and directed slightly laterally.
- Contact bone on the medial aspect of the femur (on or near the lesser trochanter).
- 'Walk off' medially and travel a further 5 cm (approximately).
- Elicit signs and inject as before.

Popliteal fossa approach

- Patient lying prone.
- point of insertion is 7 cm proximal to the flexor crease and 1 cm lateral to the midline.
- 22G short-bevel needle directed slightly cephalad.
- Nerve encountered at approximately 3 – 5 cm.
- Saphenous nerve block must be added for complete anaesthesia of the foot.

••••••••••••••••••••••••••••••••

17. HOW WOULD YOU PERFORM A COELIAC PLEXUS BLOCK?

➡ **Blocks used in chronic pain management are asked occasionally in the exam.**

The coeliac plexus surrounds the origin of the coeliac artery at the superior border of the pancreas (between T12 and L1). It is a **retroperitoneal** structure. It receives both sympathetic (preganglionic white rami) and parasympathetic nerve fibres. It is formed from the union of:

- Greater Splanchnic nerve (from the 5th to 9th thoracic sympathetic ganglia)
- Lesser Splanchnic nerve (from the 10th and 11th sympathetic ganglia)
- Least Splanchnic nerve (from the 12th sympathetic ganglia)
- Coeliac branch of the vagus nerve (parasympathetic)

The plexus lies anterior to: - T12 and L1 vertebrae
                                 - Crura of the diaphragm
                                 - Aorta

The plexus is posterior to: - Stomach
                                 - Pancreas (upper border)
                                 - Left renal vein

The plexus surrounds: - Coeliac artery
                                 - Superior mesenteric artery

A standard technique for coeliac plexus block is:

- Patient lying prone on an X-ray table.
- Abdomen supported by one or two pillows to prevent lordosis of the lumbar spine.
- Locate the spinous process of the 12th thoracic vertebra (this lies over the body of L1).
- Mark a point 8 cm lateral to the midline at this level (this is at the lower border of the 12th rib).
- Direct the needle slightly cephalad and at an angle of 45 - 55° to the coronal plane.
- Missing the transverse process of L1, strike the body of the vertebra.
- Redirect slightly steeper and slide just anterior to the vertebral body.
- Final needle position is 1 - 2 cm anterior to the L1 vertebral body on the lateral film and within the vertebral body on the anteroposterior film (medial edge of the pedicle).
- X-ray opaque dye is used to confirm the correct position. It should spread up and down in a narrow band.
- Injection of the chosen solution follows careful and regular **aspiration**.
- Bilateral block is required.

Suitable solutions for temporary block are 1% lignocaine or 0.25% bupivacaine (approximately 20 ml each side is required). For permanent block, 50% alcohol may be used, although local anaesthetic should be added as the injection is painful.

Potential complications are:

- Intravascular injection (many vessels in the area i.e. aorta, vena cava, renal vein)
- Intraperitoneal injection
- Retroperitoneal haematoma
- Backache
- Hypotension (particularly orthostatic)
- Neuritis
- Impotence

....

18. WHAT ANATOMICAL STRUCTURES ARE ENCOUNTERED DURING SPINAL ANAESTHESIA?

➡ **This should be fundamental anatomical knowledge for the anaesthetist.**

The spinal cord ends at the level of L1,2 in the adult (L3,4 in the child). When answering the question you must state the level at which you are performing the procedure. The structures traversed at L3,4 (from superficial to deep) are:

- Skin and subcutaneous tissue.
- Supraspinous ligament – joins the tips of the spinous processes of the vertebrae.
- Interspinous ligament – thin ligament between the spinous processes.
- Ligamentum flavum – runs from lamina above to the one below.
- Extradural space – contains extradural fat and the venous plexus.
- Dura mater – longitudinal fibres.
- Subdural space – only a potential space between the dura and arachnoid maters.
- Arachnoid mater – thin layer only.
- Subarachnoid space – contains the CSF, the cauda equina (leash of nerve roots) and the filum terminale (the prolongation of the spinal pia mater).

If the needle continued anteriorly, it would pass through the dural layers and the posterior longitudinal ligament before hitting the body of the vertebra (or intervertebral disc).

....

19. HOW DO YOU PERFORM A CAUDAL BLOCK?

➡ **It is important to remember which structures extend into the sacral canal, especially when using the block in children.**

The sacral canal curves with the sacrum and is triangular in cross section. It is closed anteriorly and posteriorly by the fused masses of the five sacral vertebrae. The nerves running in the sacral canal exit via the anterior and posterior sacral foraminae (four on each side). The nerves exiting via the anterior foraminae gain access to the pelvis, while those passing through the posterior foraminae enter the erector spinae muscles on the posterior surface of the sacrum. Failure of fusion of the laminae of the 5th (and often the 4th) sacral vertebra leaves a hiatus (**the sacral hiatus**). The sacral hiatus, flanked on either side by the sacral cornua, provides inferior access to the canal. It is covered by the sacro-coccygeal ligament. The 5th sacral nerve, the coccygeal nerves and the filum terminale pierce the arachnoid and dura mater at S2,3 and exit via the sacral hiatus.

The following structures are found in the sacral canal:

- Cauda equina
- Filum terminale
- Spinal meninges (with CSF in the subarachnoid space down to the level of S2,3)
- Sacral and coccygeal nerves (5 pairs of each)
- Epidural venous plexus (and lymphatics)
- Epidural fat

A standard technique for caudal block is:

- Patient in the lateral position (prone also used).
- Head, shoulders and ankles supported to avoid pelvic tilt.
- Knees drawn up in front of the abdomen.
- Locate the hiatus between the sacral cornua (the apex of an equilateral triangle with its base on a line joining the posterior superior iliac spines points to the hiatus).
- Insert a 20G needle, at 45° to the skin, until it just passes through the sacro-coccygeal ligament.
- Advancement within the canal is not necessary and increases the risk of problems.
- Injection follows careful and regular aspiration for blood and CSF.

In adults a volume of 20 ml of local anaesthetic is required.

In the child, caudal block can provide excellent analgesia up to the level of the umbilicus (T10). The greater spread of anaesthetic in the child is attributed to the loosely packed epidural fat and the lack of dense fibrous bands between the fat lobules. In most cases, the sacral cornua are easy to feel in the child. However, with the hips flexed to 90°, the cornua normally lie on the line of the long axis of the femur. Suitable volumes of local anaesthetic in the child are shown in the table below. The author uses bupivacaine 0.25% for volumes < 20 ml and bupivacaine 0.19% if > 20 ml.

Level of block required	Volume (ml kg⁻¹)
Sacral / Lower lumbar (i.e. perineal surgery)	0.5
Lumbar (i.e. hernia surgery)	1.0
Lower thoracic (i.e. testicular surgery)	1.25

....

5 QUESTIONS ON SAFETY

1. WHY IS A CAPNOGRAM SO USEFUL?

➡ **This is all about airway safety.**

The Report of the Confidential Enquiries into Maternal Deaths in the United Kingdom 1988-1990 states:

"It is recommended that a CO_2 analyser should be provided in all locations where a general anaesthetic is administered."

It is significant that, in this report, there were four deaths directly attributable to anaesthesia, and one late death attributable; of the five, four were due to airway difficulties.

Similarly, airway mismanagement contributes to morbidity and mortality in the general surgical population. In the Report of the National Confidential Enquiry into Perioperative Deaths 1991/1992, capnography was used in 1113 of 1616 deaths in theatre but in only 166 cases at induction. The report goes on to say:

"Expired CO_2 analysis is one, although not the only, means whereby satisfactory airway management can be assured and its use may save lives."

The use of capnography as a routine measure is recommended by both the American Society of Anaesthetists and the Association of Anaesthetists of Great Britain and Ireland:

"A pulse oximeter and capnometer must be available for every patient" (Recommendations for Standards of Monitoring during Anaesthesia and Recovery 1994).

••••••••••••••••••••••••••••••

2. HOW CAN A PATIENT'S TEMPERATURE BE MAINTAINED DURING THE COURSE OF A LONG OPERATION?

➡ **The human is a homeotherm, with enzymatic, cerebral and muscular activity all depending on body temperature staying within the limits of 34-42°C. Postoperative hypothermia has particular implications for recovery of neuromuscular function.**

Consider *attenuation of losses,* and *provision of heat*, separately.

Attenuation of heat loss:

Loss occurs by means of radiation, convection, conduction and evaporation. The head is a particular source of radiant loss, especially in the neonate. Loss through convection is increased under anaesthesia because of vasodilation, and when body cavities are open, as at laparotomy. Radiant heat loss may be reduced by the use of a reflective "space blanket" while convective loss is minimalised by keeping the patient covered, especially the head. Conductive loss is less of a problem, other than in the case of administration of large amounts of cold fluid, which is to be avoided. They should be warmed instead. Evaporative loss from body cavities and expired gases is significant, and may be reduced by the use of heat and moisture exchangers (HME) and circle breathing systems.

The isothermic saturation boundary (ISB) is the point at which gas in the bronchial tree reaches 37°C and 100% humidity; this is normally at the carina. Breathing a dry gas mixture moves the ISB downwards, so that large airways are exposed to dry gases and so participate in heat and moisture exchange. One observed effect of an HME is to restore the ISB towards the normal position.

Active heating:

Heat is generated by basal metabolism, which is reduced by anaesthesia, and by muscular activity, which is all but abolished when muscle relaxation is employed: not only are all muscles inactive, but there is no work of breathing as the patient's lungs are artificially ventilated. Means of providing active warming include:

- Maintaining ambient temperature in theatre above 22°C.
- Warming administered intravenous fluids.
- Warming blankets on operating table.
- Warming blanket in patient bed prior to transfer from operating table.

••••••••••••••••••••••••••••••

3. WHAT DEVICES IN THE ANAESTHETIC MACHINE PREVENT BAROTRAUMA?

➡ **The supply for machines in theatre is by pipeline, with cylinders as back-up. The gases are delivered at 4 Bar (420 kPa, 60 psi).**

Oxygen is stored in a Vacuum Insulated Evaporator (VIE) at -183° and nitrous oxide is stored in a manifold of cylinders. After heat exchanging and pressure reduction, gases enter the theatre at terminal outlets, where a Schrader probe leads to a gas-specific hose, which in turn connects to a Non-Interchangeable Screw Thread (NIST) at the anaesthetic machine. There are either one or two pressure regulators (also called pressure reducing valves) within the machine (the number depends on the manufacturer) after which there is a pressure relief valve which operates at 800 kPa (8 Bar, 120 psi) in order to protect the machine from damage. On the back bar, where the vaporisers are situated, there is a pressure relief valve which operates at 42 kPa (6 psi); it is this which protects the patient. The reservoir bag will also burst at less than one atmosphere.

....

4. DO YOU WEAR ANTI-STATIC SHOES?

➡ **This introduces a discussion about anti-static precautions.**

Shoes for wear in theatre no longer have to be made to anti-static standards, as these precautions are now being removed. This is because the explosive agents, ether and cyclopropane, are no longer in current usage. Where they are still used, anti-static precautions still pertain.

The purpose of anti-static measures is to *improve* the conduction of electricity to ground, so as to reduce the risk of a spark in the presence of a build-up of static. Anti-static precautions include:

- Terazzo flooring. This is made of stone, and has a very low electrical resistance, allowing current to flow to earth. It is extremely expensive to build and requires strengthened ceilings. Theatres built in future will not have terazzo flooring. Where it exists, it has a resistance of 20,000 - 500,000 Ω between two points 60 cm apart.
- Equipment in contact with the floor has carbonised rubber wheels.
- Other anaesthetic equipment which is antistatic includes facemasks, catheter mounts and breathing systems. These carry a yellow marker to indicate that they are made from carbonised rubber.
- Humidity above 50% and temperature above 20°C confers protection against the formation of sparks.
- Theatre shoes were previously manufactures with a conductive plug in the heel, to provide an electrical contact between the sole of the foot of the anaesthetist (or assistant, surgeon, or nurse) and the terazzo floor.

....

5. WHAT ELEMENTS ARE NEEDED FOR A FIRE?

➡ **A fire is the result of the reaction of a combustible agent with an oxidising agent that proceeds releasing energy as heat and light.**

It should be noted that despite the withdrawal of flammable anaesthetic agents from use in the UK the risk of fire or explosion in theatres is still present and the examiners will still expect you to know about it (examples include explosions due to methane in bowel gas, spillage of cleaning fluids, especially ether and during laser surgery).

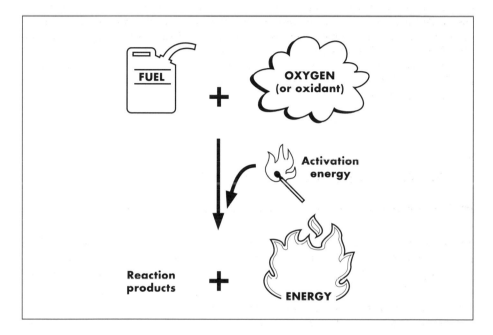

The reaction between the combustible agent (the fuel) and the oxidising agent (commonly but not exclusively oxygen) is started by when a small amount of energy is provided to act as a activator (the activation energy). However once the reaction is under way the heat energy that results from it is often enough to sustain the fire in a self-propagating manner.

• •

6. WHAT SAFETY FEATURES AND PRACTICES ARE IMPORTANT IN USING GAS CYLINDERS?

➡ **These may be divided into storage, identification, testing and connection.**

Storage

A. Large cylinders should be stored upright, whilst smaller ones and importantly Entonox must be stored horizontally.

B. They should be kept indoors and protected from weather and extremes of temperature.

C. By using the cylinders in rotation the use of each cylinder is similar to that of all the others. This ensures that the interval between testing is appropriate.

D. Medical gases are stored separately from other gases and in the past when flammable gases were used these were stored separately from other medical gases.

E. The cylinders are made of manganese steel, high carbon steel or aluminium alloy to ensure that they are able to resist the high internal pressures. (Cylinders should be able to withstand approximately 170% of their maximum working pressure). It should be noted that even these materials do not stop the risk of explosion if the cylinder is dropped on a hard surface.

Identification

A. Cylinders may be identified by their colour coding and the system used in the UK is the international standard of colours for medical gases (ISO/R32). It should be noted that this standard despite being international is NOT world-wide (e.g. oxygen cylinders in the UK are black with white shoulders, but in the USA they are green and in Germany blue with white shoulders).

B. They are stamped with the owners mark (normally the gas supply company), a serial number, the testing pressure as well as a mark that records the pressure testing (see below). They are also stamped with a safe filling pressure.

C. Cylinders also have clearly written labels permanently attached. This also contains information on the safety precautions required for use (particularly the avoidance of oil on cylinders of gases that support combustion (oxygen, Entonox and nitrous oxide).

Testing

A. Medical cylinders are regularly inspected and tested by the manufacturers including endoscopic internal examination. Also one of each batch is tested to destruction during manufacture so the quality of the metal used for manufacture is ensured. Faulty cylinders are destroyed.

B. Cylinders in the UK have a plastic disc inserted between the valve and the body, the colour and shape of which is determined by the date of the last examination.

Connection

A. The cylinders that we use in theatre have a pin-index system on their valve bodies to ensure that accidental connection to the wrong yoke cannot occur. (Though there are a number of way in which the pin-index system can be deliberately overcome, including using three Bodek seals or filing off one of the pins).

B. Before attaching a new cylinder it is advisable to open the cylinder momentarily to blow out any dust that is lodged in the outlet of the cylinder to stop this entering the anaesthetic machine and its circuits.

C. The cylinder should be turned on slowly to reduce the risk of adiabatic heating due to a rapid increase in pressure within the machine. The cylinder should be turned on fully to reduce the fall of pressure as the cylinder empties. When turning off the cylinder this should be done with only moderate force in order minimise damage to the valve seating.

....

7. WHY IS A PATIENT NOT ELECTROCUTED BY DIATHERMY?

The effects of an alternating current on tissues is related to the current density (current per unit area). High currents are focused onto small areas to cause the local burning that is the object of diathermy. However in order to be of a threat to the patient (not by burning him) the current must depolarise excitable tissue (nerves and muscle). It is this excitation of tissue that causes ventricular fibrillation. The susceptibility of the tissue to current is related to the frequency applied. If the frequency is between 40 and 60 Hz then the required current for ventricular fibrillation is small, and if applied directly to the heart is very small indeed (approximately 150 μA), however as the frequency is increased tissue becomes less and less susceptible to excitation, and at the frequencies used for diathermy (1 to 1.5 MHz) there is little muscle excitation even at currents high enough to cause burning.

....

8. WHAT FACTORS PREDISPOSE TO NERVE INJURY DURING ANAESTHESIA, GIVING EXAMPLES?

➡ **Nerve injury occurs either because the nerve becomes ischaemic or is directly traumatised. Ischaemia may be caused by compression or excessive stretching.**

Direct trauma

A. Occurs during regional anaesthesia. It is due to either damage to the nerve by the needle itself or to intraneuronal injection of local anaesthetic. The latter causes a local pressure effect and therefore local ischaemia. It can be minimised by performing the block with the patient awake as the intraneuronal injection is ´extremely painful and the patient will be able to warn the anaesthetist. Needle damage is said to be reduced by the use of atraumatic short-bevelled needles that are not designed to cut tissue and by the use of nerve stimulators rather than paraesthesia to ascertain needle placement.

B. Direct chemical trauma is the result of injection of neurotoxic agents around the nerve. This may be intentional (phenol is used to damage nerves in the treatment of chronic pain) or accidental. The latter risk is minimised by careful checking of all drugs used during regional anaesthesia.

Ischaemic Damage

A. Poor positioning of the patient may cause prolonged compression or stretching of nerves.

B. Tourniquets are commonly associated with nerve injuries especially the radial nerve. It is recommended that the tourniquet is only used for 2 hours (with an absolute maximum of 3 hours).

C. Causes of poor perfusion (e.g. hypotension) or microvascular dysfunction (diabetes) are associated with ischaemic nerve damage.

D. Muscle relaxation allow overstretching of nerves.

The most common area of damage is the brachial plexus. It is generally damaged by poor positioning either by stretching from lateral flexion of the neck or from excessive abduction of the arm. It may also be compressed in the prone position by compression between the clavicle and first rib. Trendelenburg positioning with a shoulder brace was a common cause of brachial plexus injury before non–slip operating tables were produced.

Other nerves injured include:

A. *Ulna nerve* – as it passes superficially on the lateral aspect of the elbow

B. *Radial nerve* – as it passes through the spiral groove it may be damaged by the arm hanging with the upper arm pressing against the table edge. It may also be damaged distally during radial arterial cannulation.

C. *Common peroneal nerve* - as it winds around the head of the fibula (analogous to the ulna nerve in the arm).

D. *Sciatic and femoral nerves* - may be damaged by excessive angulation or rotation of the hips, the latter nerve specifically in the lithotomy position.

E. *Facial nerves* - may be damaged by direct pressure around the eyes or on the cheeks when the patient is placed in the prone position.

....

9. WHAT IS THE STOICHIOMETRIC CONCENTRATION AND THE FLAMMABILITY LIMITS OF A MIXTURE?

➡ **The stoichiometric concentration is that relative concentration of the mixture of combustible agent (as vapour) and oxidising agent at which the reaction that occurs uses up all the available agents.**

It is the concentration that the most complete reaction can happen for a given volume of combustible agent, and so it is the most violent reaction. If the reaction is so intense that it can spread within the mixture at a speed that is faster than the speed of sound then an explosion occurs.

If the proportions are allowed to differ more and more from this ideal the intensity of the reaction is reduced until the disproportion is so great that the reaction cannot start. This limit (and there are both an upper and a lower limit) is called the flammability limit.

An example would be ether:

	Lower flammability limit	Stoichiometric concentration	Upper flammability limit
Ether & Air	2%	3.4%	34%
Ether & Oxygen	2%	14%	82%

Obviously in oxygen (as opposed to air) there is a greater presence of oxidising agent and there is absence of nitrogen. The nitrogen acts by inhibiting the reaction, diluting the constituents and by absorbing some of the energy released. In general the risk of a reaction violent enough to case an explosion with vapours seen in anaesthetic practice is only present if the oxygen concentration is greater than that in room air.

....

10. WHAT METHODS ARE AVAILABLE ON THE STANDARD ANAESTHETIC MACHINE TO STOP THE DELIVERY OF A HYPOXIC GAS MIXTURE?

➡ **As with most questions that relate to the flow of gas through the machine or through a circuit the best way of dealing with this is to start at the wall and follow the gas flow through the machine to the patient.**

1. Although the provision of the piped medical gases is not the responsibility of the anaesthetist it should be noted that there are specific regulations that control this supply, and its maintenance (HTM 22 in the UK).

2. The wall fitting for pipeline supply consists of a Schrader socket with an indexed collar. The socket is fixed to the flexible hose, and can only be removed by   a service engineer. It is also designed so it cannot be attached to the wrong hose by accident. This is then permanently attached to the hose with a stainless steel ferrule.

3. The flexible non-compressible hose is colour coded along its whole length to prevent accidental mis-connection if the hose is shortened. Although there are cases of cross-connection or errors in manufacturing (connecting the oxygen socket to the blue nitrous oxide hose) these have generally been minimised by tighter quality control and separation of the different assembly lines during manufacturing.

4. The machine end of the hose is permanently attached to a non-interchangeable connection consisting of a probe with gas-specific sized shoulders and a nut that can be connected to the machine with a spanner (known as a 'NIST', non-interchangeable screw threaded, connection).

5. Methods to ensure the correct connection of the cylinder supply including the pin-index system are discussed elsewhere it the book. (*see* – ***What safety features and practices are important in using gas cylinders?***)

6. The risk of leakage within the machine pipework is minimised by using gas-tight connections, either compression fittings (similar to domestic plumbing fittings), sealing washers or tapered threads.

7. Many machines feature secondary regulators that reduce the pressure within the machine to just below pipeline pressure (420 kPa) so that any fluctuation in the pipeline pressure (e.g. due to demand) is smoothed out.

8. The flowmeter bank on UK anaesthetic machines has to conform to BS 4272, so that the knobs must be labelled with the gas that they control, and the oxygen knob must be uniquely octagonal in profile, it must be the largest and must project more than 2 mm proud of the other knobs. The oxygen knob is furthermore always placed on the left.

9. The flowmeters themselves have a number of features that help ensure accuracy, and so avoid the delivery of a hypoxic mixture. The bobbin has fins cut into its upper surface to make it spin, and so reduce the risk of sticking. There is also a conductive strip or coating on the inside of the tube to reduce the build-up of electrostatic charges and this also helps minimise sticking. Furthermore the tubes are so designed that the bobbin cannot be hidden at the top of the tube.

10. Many machines now have an anti-hypoxia device linked to the flowmeters. The most commonly seen of these is the Ohmeda Link 25, that is a mechanical connection between the oxygen and nitrous oxide flowmeter knobs that ensures that it is impossible to dial a nitrous oxide : oxygen ratio of more than 3:1 (i.e. an oxygen of 25%). This does not however consider any of the other gases attached or changes in the supply pressure.

11. Machines are fitted with an oxygen failure device (see *How does an oxygen disconnect alarm work?*)

12. Despite the left placement of the oxygen flowmeter, there is a risk of hypoxic delivery if there is a crack in one of the other flowmeters if the oxygen flows into the back bar on the left, before the inflow of the other gases. Therefore the gas from the oxygen flowmeter is ducted so that it enters the back bar downstream of the other gases.

••••••••••••••••••••••••••••••

11. HOW DOES SaO$_2$ CHANGE AFTER VENTILATOR DISCONNECTION AND UNNOTICED OXYGEN SUPPLY FAILURE?

➡ **It should be remembered that a patient who is apnoeic will desaturate much more slowly than one who is ventilated with a hypoxic mixture.**

In the latter case the oxygen reservoir in the lungs (equal to Functional Residual Capacity (FRC) x F_AO_2) is washed out quickly and then the oxygen in the mixed venous blood may actually start to pass out of the pulmonary arteries as it passes through the lungs.

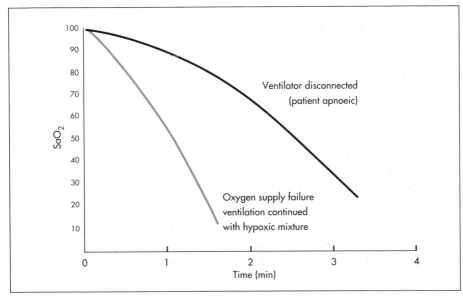

••••••••••••••••••••••••••••••

12. HOW DOES AN OXYGEN DISCONNECT ALARM WORK?

➡ Oxygen failure alarms were initially introduced when the oxygen supply was provided by cylinders to reduce the risks of hypoxia due to emptying of these cylinders. Even with the almost universal use of nearly uninterrupted pipeline supply of oxygen it is still a requirement under British Standard for anaesthetic machines to be fitted with an oxygen failure alarm.

The alarm is auditory (of at least 7 second duration and a specific minimum volume), and is powered by the oxygen supply itself to activate when the oxygen supply pressure falls to 200 kPa. It should also cut off the supply of the now hypoxic fresh gas flow from the patient and replace this with air either from an air supply or from the room.

A common oxygen failure device relies on a spring-loaded piston that is moved by the action of oxygen pressure on a diaphragm. As the supply pressure starts to fail (at 260 kPa) the piston is moved back by the spring, opening an auxiliary gas channel allowing gas to pass through the oxygen failure whistle sounding the alarm. This will continue to sound until the supply pressure fails to 40.5 kPa. As the pressure continues to fall (200 kPa) the piston moves further and finally is pulled onto a seating magnet that closes off the fresh gas flow by closing the cut-off valve. The fresh gas flow passes out through the pressure relief valve. This final movement also opens the air inspiratory valve and allow the patient (if not paralysed) to breath room air.

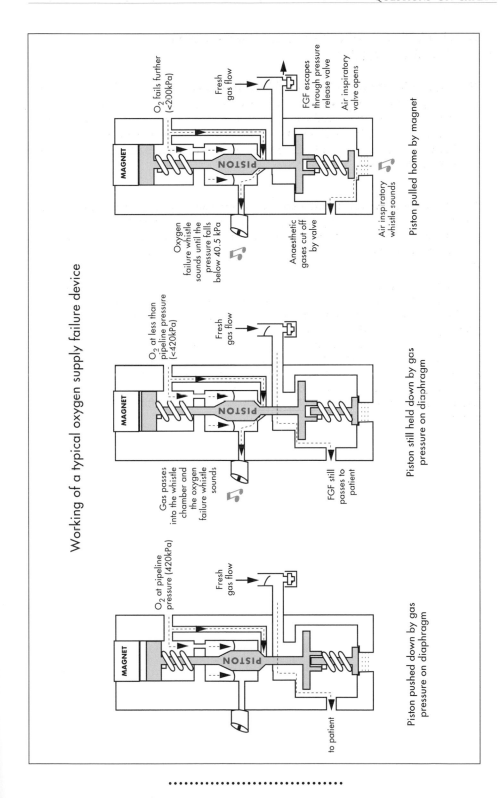

Working of a typical oxygen supply failure device

13. WHAT ARE THE COMPLICATIONS ASSOCIATED WITH A CENTRAL VENOUS CATHETER?

➡ **Most anaesthetists will perform central venous cannulation at least weekly and should have a ready list of complications of the technique.**

Direct observation of the great vessels after cannulation at, for example, thoracotomy, where the outside surface of the vessel is exposed, reveals the extent of the intimal damage that even the slickest cannulation causes. The complications of central venous cannulation may be divided into immediate and late, and include:

Immediate complications:

- Pain
- Haemorrhage: this is especially hazardous if a large bleed occurs from a subclavian approach, since the high compliance of the thoracic cavity will not constrain the bleed and a haemothorax is possible. The bleeding is not visible and pressure cannot be applied to it.
- Air embolism. The cannulation must be performed with a degree of head–down tilt.
- Cardiac arrhythmia, if the tip of the cannula lies in the atrium.
- Cardiac tamponnade, if the cannula perforates the wall of the atrium.
- Pneumothorax and subcutaneous emphysema. The needle should never be detached from the syringe while in the tissues, because if it lies inadvertently in the thoracic cavity it will allow air to enter and a pneumothorax to develop.
- Carotid artery puncture, at the internal jugular approach.
- Direct damage to adjacent structures:

  - Brachial plexus
  - Phrenic nerve
  - Thoracic duct
  - Sympathetic chain

- Misplacement: there are reports of misplacement of central venous cannulae in the thoracic cavity, the subcutaneous tissues, and even the subarachnoid space.
- Misdirection; it is not uncommon for a cannula to deviate up into the internal jugular when introduced into the subclavian vein, or across to the contralatera side.

Delayed complications:

- Sepsis
- Inconvenience (subclavian approach is better from a nursing point of view).
- Air embolism on removal, unless supine when removed.
- Embolisation of catheter fragments; for this reason, the needle should never be reintroduced into the cannula.
- Thombosis around the cannula, and subsequent embolism.
- Cardiac tamponnade, from erosion of the wall of the superior vena cava or the atrium.
- Knotting and difficulty in removal.

•••••••••••••••••••••••••••••••

14. WHAT IS THE DIFFERENCE BETWEEN DECONTAMINATION, DISINFECTION AND STERILISATION?

➡ **Although these issues appear to relate to the surgeon rather than the anaesthetist it should be remembered that reusable equipment is commonly used by anaesthetists and the methods used to ensure their safety is a fair topic for an examiner.**

Decontamination is the removal of infected material, and involves thorough cleaning and scrubbing. It makes the object more acceptable both bacteriologically and aesthetically. Detergents may be used, ranging from soap to 'Neodex'. After decontamination the object may be said to be 'clean'.

Disinfection involves the removal or killing of most of the infective organisms on the object. However there are resistant form of organisms such as spores that are NOT disabled by disinfection. It is adequate for many purposes, and avoids the use of high temperatures and pressures.

Sterilisation is the killing of all organisms including the resistant forms (spores). It may involve high temperatures and pressures, or chemical means.

It should be noted that these descriptions relate to the treatment of infectious matter, but has no indication about the removal or neutralisation of chemical contaminants.

••••••••••••••••••••••••••••••

15. HOW DO YOU PERFORM DECONTAMINATION, DISINFECTION AND STERILISATION?

➡ **Decontamination must be performed before either of the other two processes can be undertaken, as it removes the bulk of the infected material. This is important as the other procedures are only designed to be successful at treating small quantities of infected material.**

Decontamination

Decontamination may be done in a medical version of the dishwasher, or by an ultrasonic washer. Most commonly it is done by hand scrubbing in detergent and hot water, followed by rinsing and air drying.

Disinfection

Disinfection is most commonly performed by pasteurisation. This involves heating in a water bath (or in a low-pressure autoclave) and maintaining the required temperature for a set time. By not boiling plastic and rubber objects their usable life may be prolonged, as boiling tends to distort or perish them.

Temperature	Time
70°C	20 min
80°C	10 min
100°C	5 min

Boiling for a shorter period is equally successful if the object can withstand the heat.

It should be noted that the timing is from when the temperature of the water has returned to the required temperature after the last object has been inserted.

Chemical disinfection may be undertaken with 70% alcohol in water, chlorhexidine (either in 0.05% water with soaking for 30 minutes, or more rapidly by using 0.5% solution in 70% alcohol, in which case only 2 minutes is required), hypochlorite solutions ('bleach'), or gluteraldehyde.

Sterilisation

Sterilisation in theatres is most effectively and quickly performed by autoclaving. An autoclave is effectively a pressured steam cooker. The objects are placed in a gas tight chamber and steam is pumped into and around the chamber raising the temperature and pressure. The time required depends on the temperature and the pressure. Chemical markers (such as the brown stripes on the tape of sterile supply bags) help ascertain that the autoclaving has been adequate.

Pressure	Temperature	Time
15 psi	122°C	30 min
20 psi	126°C	10 min
30 psi	134°C	3 min

Rubber and plastic items may be damaged by autoclaving, or may only last for a number of cycles before they must be disposed of, and many other items are not suitable for the rigors of the process.

The other method used commonly in theatre involves gluteraldehyde (also known as 'Cydex®') which when used in adequate concentration for long enough is an effective sterilising agent.

Other techniques include low pressure steam (at less than atmospheric pressure) used for delicate items, formaldehyde and ethylene oxide which can be used to sterilise whole anaesthetic machines.

Most disposable equipment is sterilised by gamma irradiation at the manufacturer.

● ●

INDEX